Medical and Surgical Management of Ocular Surface Disease in Exotic Animals

Editor

SARAH L. CZERWINSKI

VETERINARY CLINICS
OF NORTH AMERICA:
EXOTIC ANIMAL PRACTICE

www.vetexotic.theclinics.com

Consulting Editor
JÖRG MAYER

January 2019 • Volume 22 • Number 1

ELSEVIER

1600 John F. Kennedy Boulevard • Suite 1800 • Philadelphia, Pennsylvania, 19103-2899
http://www.vetexotic.theclinics.com

VETERINARY CLINICS OF NORTH AMERICA: EXOTIC ANIMAL PRACTICE Volume 22, Number 1
January 2019 ISSN 1094-9194, ISBN-13: 978-0-323-65507-1

Editor: Colleen Dietzler
Developmental Editor: Meredith Madeira

Veterinary Clinics of North America: Exotic Animal Practice (ISSN 1094-9194) is published in January, May, and September by Elsevier, Inc., 360 Park Avenue South, New York, NY 10010-1710. Subscription prices are $284.00 per year for US individuals, $519.00 per year for US institutions, $100.00 per year for US students and residents, $338.00 per year for Canadian individuals, $626.00 per year for Canadian institutions, $352.00 per year for international individuals, $626.00 per year for international institutions and $165.00 per year for Canadian and foreign students/residents. To receive student/resident rate, orders must be accompanied by name of affiliated institution, date of term, and the *signature* of program/residency coordinator on institution letterhead. Orders will be billed at individual rate until proof of status is received. Foreign air speed delivery is included in all *Clinics* subscription prices. All prices are subject to change without notice. **POSTMASTER:** Send address changes to *Veterinary Clinics of North America: Exotic Animal Practice*, Elsevier Health Sciences Division, Subscription Customer Service, 3251 Riverport Lane, Maryland Heights, MO 63043. **Customer Service: Telephone: 1-800-654-2452** (U.S. and Canada); **1-314-447-8871** (outside U.S. and Canada). **Fax: 1-314-447-8029. E-mail: journalscustomerservice-usa@elsevier.com (for print support); journalsonlinesupport-usa@elsevier.com (for online support).**

Reprints. For copies of 100 or more of articles in this publication, please contact the Commercial Reprints Department, Elsevier Inc., 360 Park Avenue South, New York, New York 10010-1710. Tel.: 212-633-3874; Fax: 212-633-3820; E-mail: reprints@elsevier.com.

Veterinary Clinics of North America: Exotic Animal Practice is covered in *MEDLINE/PubMed (Index Medicus)*.

Contributors

CONSULTING EDITOR

JÖRG MAYER, Dr med vet, Msc
Diplomate, American Board of Veterinary Practitioners (Exotic Companion
Mammals); Diplomate, European College of Zoological Medicine (Small Mammals);
Diplomate, American College of Zoological Medicine; Associate Professor of
Zoological Medicine, Department of Small Animal Medicine and Surgery, University
of Georgia College of Veterinary Medicine, Athens, Georgia, USA

EDITOR

SARAH L. CZERWINSKI, DVM
Diplomate, American College of Veterinary Ophthalmologists; Clinical Assistant
Professor of Ophthalmology, Department of Small Animal Medicine and Surgery,
University of Georgia Veterinary Teaching Hospital, Athens, Georgia, USA

AUTHORS

KATHLEEN M. BEDARD, DVM
Resident, Comparative Ophthalmology, University of Georgia, Athens, Georgia,
USA

CARMEN MARIA HELENA COLITZ, DVM, PhD
Diplomate, American College of Veterinary Ophthalmologists; Owner, All Animal Eye
Care, Inc, Jupiter, Florida; Adjunct Faculty Member, Department of Molecular
Biomedical Sciences, North Carolina State University, Raleigh, North Carolina,
USA

SARAH L. CZERWINSKI, DVM
Diplomate, American College of Veterinary Ophthalmologists; Clinical Assistant
Professor of Ophthalmology, Department of Small Animal Medicine and Surgery,
University of Georgia Veterinary Teaching Hospital, Athens, Georgia, USA

NICOLA DI GIROLAMO, DMV, GPCert (ExAP), MSc (EBHC), PhD
Diplomate, European College of Zoological Medicine (Herpetology); Tai Wai Small Animal
& Exotic Hospital, Tai Wai, Shatin, Hong Kong

ANGELA GRIGGS, DVM
Diplomate, American College of Veterinary Ophthalmologists; Private Practice, North
Houston Veterinary Ophthalmology, Spring, Texas, USA

CAROLINE MONK, DVM
Diplomate, American College of Veterinary Ophthalmologists; Associate Veterinarian,
Ophthalmology, BluePearl Veterinary Partners, Atlanta, Georgia, USA

KATHERN E. MYRNA, DVM, MS
Diplomate, American College of Veterinary Ophthalmologists; Associate Professor of Ophthalmology, Department of Small Animal Medicine and Surgery, UGA Veterinary Medical Center, University of Georgia, Athens, Georgia, USA

KATHRYN M. SMITH FLEMING, DVM, PhD
Diplomate, American College of Veterinary Ophthalmologists; Assistant Professor of Ophthalmology, Department of Veterinary Clinical Medicine, University of Illinois at Urbana-Champaign, Urbana, Illinois, USA

DAVID L. WILLIAMS, MA, MEd, VetMD, PhD, CertVOphthal, CertWEL, FHEA, FRCVS
Diplomate, European College of Animal Welfare and Behaviour Medicine; Department of Veterinary Medicine, University of Cambridge, Cambridge, United Kingdom

Contents

VETERINARY CLINICS OF NORTH AMERICA: EXOTIC ANIMAL PRACTICE

SERIES OF RELATED INTEREST

Veterinary Clinics of North America: Small Animal Practice
Available at: https://www.vetsmall.theclinics.com/

THE CLINICS ARE NOW AVAILABLE ONLINE!
Access your subscription at:
www.theclinics.com

Preface

Introduction to Ocular Surface Disease in Exotics

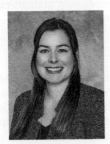

Sarah L. Czerwinski, DVM, DACVO
Editor

The ocular surface is made up of the precorneal tear film, the conjunctiva, and the cornea, forming the first part of the visual pathway. The clear cornea allows light to pass through so that the photoreceptors in the retina can be stimulated, allowing the brain to perceive images. For land animals, the tear film in conjunction with the cornea forms a significant refractive structure of the eye. The conjunctiva and precorneal tear film are essential for preventing infection and preserving the integrity of the cornea.

PRECORNEAL TEAR FILM

The precorneal tear film plays an important role in the ocular defense system. It prevents desiccation of the conjunctival and corneal surface, irrigates the ocular surface to remove debris, and contains enzymes, proteins, and immunoglobulins. Depending on the species, the tear film is made up of lipid, aqueous, and mucus components.

Tear production is quantified in millimeters per minute using a Schirmer tear test strip placed in the lower eyelid. Because of the relatively large size of this strip and the small size of the palpebral fissure and low tear volume in many exotic species, alternative methods, including the phenol red thread test and the paper point tear test, were developed.

The nasolacrimal drainage system varies greatly between species and may be a common source of disease.

CONJUNCTIVA

The conjunctiva consists of connective tissue and overlying epithelium that covers the sclera from the limbus, forms the fornix, and covers the bulbar surface of the upper and

Vet Clin Exot Anim 22 (2019) ix–x
https://doi.org/10.1016/j.cvex.2018.09.002
1094-9194/19/© 2018 Published by Elsevier Inc.

lower eyelids as well as the nictitans. It is a critical part of the mucosal immune system and is normally inhabited by commensal organisms.

CORNEA

The cornea is essentially a modification of the sclera to form a "window" through which light can pass into the eye. Depending on the species, it may contain an anterior epithelium, stroma, and posterior epithelium (endothelium) containing sodium-potassium ATPase pumps that assist in maintaining corneal deturgescence.

CHALLENGES IN EXOTIC SPECIES

Ocular surface disease is relatively common overall, in part due to the necessary exposure of the cornea and the challenges presented by the required absence of a direct vascular supply. Diagnosis and therapy for ocular surface disease in exotic animals present several challenges: there is a relative paucity of literature about many of these species compared with domestic animals; anatomic and environmental variations can contribute to the pathogenesis and management of disease. The following articles review the diagnosis and treatment of ocular surface disease in several species of exotic animals.

Sarah L. Czerwinski, DVM, DACVO
Department of Small Animal Medicine
and Surgery
University of Georgia
Veterinary Teaching Hospital
2200 College Station Road
Athens, GA 30602, USA

E-mail address:
Sarah.Czerwinski@uga.edu

Ocular Surface Disease of Rabbits

Kathleen M. Bedard, DVM

KEYWORDS

- Rabbit • Cornea • Conjunctiva • Dacryocystitis • Surface disease

KEY POINTS

- The prominent, laterally placed eyes of the rabbit predispose it to surface injury.
- The tortuous path of the nasolacrimal duct makes the rabbit prone to obstruction and subsequent inflammation and infection.
- Conjunctivitis is a common problem in the rabbit and can be due to both infectious and noninfectious (husbandry-related) causes.
- Corneal ulceration in the rabbit can be managed similarly to ulceration in canine and feline species.

INTRODUCTION

The domestic rabbit (Oryctolagus cuniculus) continues to grow in popularity as a companion animal and thus is encountered with increasing frequency by the veterinarian in private practice. Ocular problems have been reported in both populations of research and pet animals and can greatly affect quality of life and welfare. One study of 1000 pet rabbits in the United Kingdom found 26% to have ocular lesions, with 2.5% suffering from corneal lesions and another 3.5% afflicted with dacryocystitis.[1] Understanding the unique attributes of the rabbit eye and the diseases that commonly affect the eye is important to being able to treat these animals effectively. This review focuses on diseases that affect the surface of the eye, namely corneal and adnexal disease.

ANATOMY

The first detailed text describing the anatomy of the rabbit was published in 1954 by Prince.[1] Rabbits have prominent, laterally placed eyes to help facilitate nearly 360° of visualization of their environment. While enabling rabbits to better keep a look out for predators, the prominence and position of the eye leaves it exposed and subject to

Disclosure Statement: The authors have nothing to disclose.
Comparative Ophthalmology, University of Georgia, 2200 College Station Road, Athens, GA 30202, USA
E-mail address: kmbedard@uga.edu

trauma. In addition, the corneal surface is large compared with the size of the eye itself, predisposing the rabbit to ulceration.[1–4]

The rabbit has a unique nasolacrimal system in that there is only one slitlike inferior punctum, located deep within the inferior medial fornix, and no lacrimal sac.[3–5] In addition to these unique attributes, the rabbit nasolacrimal system follows a particularly tortuous route through the nasal ostium with 2 sharp diversions and areas of narrowing. This tortuous route makes them highly susceptible to developing obstructions of the duct. Finally, the nasolacrimal duct passes very close to the molar and incisor tooth roots and can easily be affected by dental disease.

The rabbit third eyelid contains no muscles, but instead is passively drawn across the eye by the action of the retractor oculi muscle, which can advance the third eyelid more than two-thirds of the way across the ocular surface.[4]

The rabbit has a circular pupil and, in nonalbino species, a highly pigmented iris. Rabbits have a very complex vascular anatomy with a large retrobulbar venous plexus. They also boast an impressive collection of tear glands, which occupy a large portion of the retrobulbar space. Finally, rabbits have a merangiotic fundus, meaning that retinal vessels extend from the optic disc along with myelinated nerve fibers to course horizontally across the back of the eye. Their visual streak is located parallel and inferior to the retinal vessels and myelin, supplied solely by the choroidal vasculature.[1,4,5]

BLEPHARITIS

Blepharitis can be caused by a variety of infectious, inflammatory, and neoplastic causes (**Fig. 1**). Diagnostic workup should include cytology, culture, and/or biopsy if indicated. One of the most common causes of infectious blepharitis in the rabbit is infection with *Treponema cuniculi*. Infection with *T cuniculi* is thought to be transmitted to neonates by the genitally infected dam.[6] Experimentally, rabbits of infected dams birthed via hysterectomy failed to develop spirochaetosis, whereas rabbits born from infected dams developed infection regardless of whether or not they were nursed from the infected dams or were fostered with noninfected dams. The diagnosis is best made by identifying the spirochete organism on conjunctival cytology. Treatment involves 3 injections of penicillin G at 40,000 IU/kg given 1 week apart. Care must be

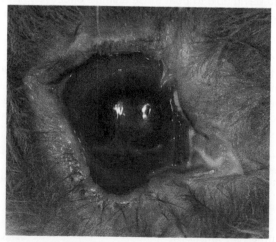

Fig. 1. Blepharitis and chronic keratitis.

used when administering systemic antibiotics to rabbits because fatal dysbiosis has been reported.[7]

Other differentials for rabbit blepharitis include myxomatosis (described further under conjunctivitis), staphylococcal infection, and squamous cell carcinoma.

NASOLACRIMAL DISEASE

Disease of the nasolacrimal duct is one of the most frequently reported ocular diseases in rabbits. In a clinical study of 344 rabbits at the University of California, Davis found that 10% of all disease presentations were ocular related and of those, 73% had clinical signs of dacryocystitis.[8] Another study of pet rabbits in 2006 found that 7 out of the 102 rabbits examined had a history of dacryocystitis.[9] Prevalence of dacryocystitis in pet rabbits in the United Kingdom has been reported to be as high as 3.5%.[1]

Dacryocystitis, or inflammation of the lacrimal sac, is diagnosed when purulent material can be expressed from the nasolacrimal puncta on placing pressure on the skin beneath the medial canthus.[8,10] However, the normal tear secretion from the gland of the third eyelid can seem milky in appearance and should therefore not be mistaken for infection.[11] In severe cases of dacryocystitis, the lacrimal gland can actually be visually distended with pus.[10] Other concurrent clinical findings can include conjunctivitis, corneal edema, and keratitis (presumably related to the presence of chronic purulent discharge on the cornea) (**Fig. 2**).

As mentioned earlier, the unique anatomy of the rabbit likely contributes the frequency of nasolacrimal duct disorders. The pathway is quite tortuous and the duct must narrow as it passes through the lacrimal to frontal bone and again at the base of the maxillary incisor (**Fig. 3**).[11] Inflammation of the nasolacrimal duct is known to cause alteration of the tear film, which becomes viscous and gritty and can block the duct at its 2 narrowest points. In addition, the duct passes quite close to both molar and incisor tooth roots.[1,3,4] Any elongation of the incisor tooth root can result in subsequent functional obstruction of the duct, and tooth root abscessation can extend locally to affect the duct as well. Blockage of the duct and stasis of the mucopurulent discharge can then lead to secondary bacterial infection.[12] In a retrospective study of 28 rabbits with dacryocystitis, 50% of cases had underlying dental disease,[10]

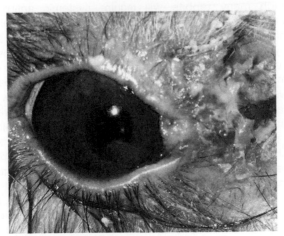

Fig. 2. Dacryocystitis and concurrent superficial corneal ulceration. (*Courtesy of* Mary Landis, VMD, MA; Whitehall PA.)

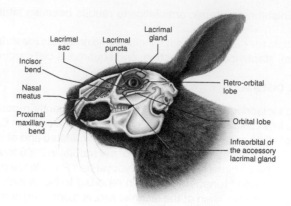

Fig. 3. Rabbit nasolacrimal duct anatomy.

making thorough oral examinations paramount in the diagnosis of nasolacrimal disease.

Primary bacterial dacryocystitis has been reported, and historically it has been most attributed to infections with *Pasteurella sp.*[11] More recent investigations have found a plethora of other bacterial agents such as *Staphylococcus sp*, *Moraxella sp*, *Oligella urethralis*, *Pseudomonas*, and *Streptococcus viridans*. However, these bacterial isolates have been found on both healthy and diseased patients, so careful interpretation of bacteriological sampling results is important.

Clinical workup of dacryocystitis should include microbiological sampling via culture and cytology of ocular discharge, Jones test, flushing of the nasolacrimal duct, complete oral examination, and skull or dental radiographs if indicated. Advanced imaging via computed tomography or dacryocystorhinography may also be indicated to identify the site of obstruction if present.

Treatment of dacryocystitis can be protracted and quite frustrating. A retrospective analysis of 28 cases of dacryocystitis in rabbits reported 5.8 weeks as the mean duration of therapy, although rabbits in this study whose disease was cured tended to have a shorter course of treatment.[10] Topical antibiotic therapy is often the first choice of treatment, although many rabbits will require systemic antibiotic therapy as well. Oral antiinflammatory agents are often indicated to help with pain and inflammation. Nasolacrimal flushing is also a mainstay of treatment, either with sterile saline, antibiotics, acetylcysteine, or some combination of these.[10] Those rabbits with underlying malocclusion or other dental disease should be treated for such if the associated nasolacrimal duct inflammation is to be resolved. Many cases will not resolve regardless of how aggressive the therapy instituted. One of the few studies looking at outcome of dacryocystitis cases indicates that the longer the treatment course, the poorer the outcome. In addition, those rabbits placed on systemic antibiotic therapy (presumably because of more severe disease) also had poorer outcomes.[10]

Finally, although congenital nasolacrimal duct obstruction in the rabbit has not been reported in the literature, rabbits have been used in studies investigating treatment of this condition because their nasolacrimal duct is structurally and histologically similar to that of people. In a study by Goldstein and colleagues[13] in 2006, balloon dacryoplasty with inflation up to 3 mm in infant New Zealand White rabbits did not induce significant inflammation or crush injury to the nasolacrimal duct. Results of this study indicate that balloon dacryoplasty could be used safely to treat congenital nasolacrimal duct obstruction if identified in a clinical setting.

NASOLACRIMAL FLUSHING

When approaching diagnostic and or therapeutic flushing of the nasolacrimal duct in cases of dacryocystitis, it is important to remember that the duct will be irritated and fragile.[11] Using rigid metal cannulas is therefore discouraged, because these can potentially perforate through the wall of the duct. Instead, soft Teflon catheters (27G) are preferred and should be introduced into the nasolacrimal puncta carefully to avoid causing trauma (**Fig. 4**). Rupture of the lacrimal sac can occur and can be identified by progressive exophthalmos when instilling irrigation fluid through the catheter, which then enters the periorbital tissue through the rent. The cornea can also easily become scratched or ulcerated during this process, so care should be taken to avoid contacting the cornea if possible.[11]

Flushing can be accomplished in the awake animal, but sedation is recommended to reduce stress in the patient and increase compliance. When flushing both eyes, a new catheter should be used for each to avoid spreading of infectious organisms. The lacrimal punctum is located deep within the ventromedial fornix of the lower eyelid. Gentle pressure can be applied to evert the lower eyelid, causing the lips of the puncta to pouch outward, allowing easy cannulation. Once the nasolacrimal punctum has been carefully catheterized, warm sterile saline or water in a 3 mL syringe can be attached to the hub and used to flush the duct. Flush can be pushed in short gentle bursts as the cannula is gently moved back and forth to try and unblock the duct. Daily or multiple flushes per week are often required to clear serious infections.

KERATOCONJUNCTIVITIS SICCA

Rabbits have 5 different tear glands that contribute to the precorneal ocular tear film: the Harderian, nictitating, lacrimal, infraorbital, and extraorbital glands.[1,3,5,14] These glands occupy a large portion of the retrobulbar space and thus disease affecting anyone of them can lead to exophthalmos. As with canine patients, rabbits can

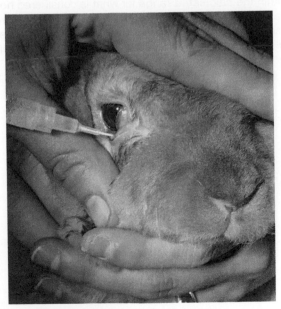

Fig. 4. Nasolacimral duct flush in a rabbit with dacryocystitis.

experience prolapse of the nictitating gland requiring surgical replacement via similar methods to improve cosmesis and avoid the development of clinical dry eye (**Fig. 5**).[4] The tear film in the rabbit is remarkably stable, which is likely why rabbits can have such a low blink rate of 3 to 4 times per hour without any associated corneal drying.[15] The normal tear osmolarity in the rabbit is between 300 and 305 mOsm/L,[16] and normal tear film breakup time has been determined to be around 20 seconds.[17]

Traditionally, clinical measurement of tear production in our domestic species is accomplished through the Schirmer tear test (STT). Measurements of normal tear production in rabbits using this method have been reported as anywhere from 5.2 to 7.6 mm/min.[18–20] Because using STT strips in smaller rabbit breeds with comparatively smaller eye size can be irritating and potentially damaging to the ocular surface, alternative tear testing to the STT has been investigated. Phenol red thread testing is better suited to measuring tear production in smaller eyes and in animals with lower tear production.[20] The test involves using a special cotton thread impregnated with phenol red, a pH-sensitive indicator that changes color from yellow to red when wetted with tears. A thread 70 mm long is crimped at one end and then placed in the ventral conjunctival fornix for 15 seconds, and the wetted length is then measured in millimeters.[21] Mean reported tear production measurements in New Zealand White rabbits using the phenol red thread test was 20.88 mm per 15 seconds with a range from 15 to 27 mm per 15 seconds.[20]

Paper point tear testing (PPTT) in rabbits is another alternative to traditional STT strips and like the phenol red thread test, avoids the ocular irritation and difficulty of inserting the large STT strip into conjunctival fornix of young dwarf breeds. Tear production in rabbits as measured by PPTT was reported to be 13.8 ± 1.5 mm/min. Investigators noted discomfort, restlessness, and a desire to try and remove the strip when using the traditional STT testing but failed to note any such behavior with the PPTT.[18]

No matter the method used to measure tear production, it is important to remember that tear production can vary between rabbit breeds, although the differences noted have still been within the calculated range for what is considered normal.[22]

Although clinical cases of keratoconjunctivitis sicca in the rabbit are rare, the rabbit has been used frequently as a model for human dry eye disease. In experimental settings, clinical dry eye in rabbits has been simulated via multiple different methods,

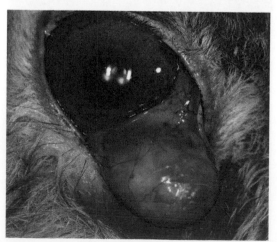

Fig. 5. Prolapsed Harderian gland. (*Courtesy of* John Sapienza, DVM, DACVO; Plainview NY.)

including giving lymphocytes sensitized to lacrimal antigens or following intralacrimal injections of concanavalin A.[23,24] Following induction of disease, the rabbit is then often used to determine the efficacy of different tear stimulants and antiinflammatories for the amelioration of clinical signs. Based on studies such as these, we know that rabbits will respond to topical treatment with 0.05% cyclosporine A after several weeks[25] and will also benefit from treatment with topical dexamethasone.[24] These findings indicate that traditional treatment of dry eye disease in other species can be successfully applied to the rabbit, should the rare clinical case of dry eye disease be presented.

Although spontaneously occurring dry eye disease is rare in the domestic rabbit, iatrogenic dry eye has been documented in rabbits experimentally treated with trimethoprim-sulfamethoxazole (TMS). Rabbits treated with 40 mg/kg of TMS by mouth twice daily demonstrated a drop in tear production by about 50% at the end of the 2-week study period.[26] Therefore, as with canine patients, rabbits treated with oral TMS should be monitored closely for any decrease in tear production.

CONJUNCTIVITIS

Conjunctivitis is a frequently encountered problem of domestic rabbits. As with other species, underlying causes of conjunctival inflammation can be mechanical (hay dust or other irritants), infectious (bacterial, fungal, viral, etc.), immune mediated (keratoconjunctivitis sicca), or neoplastic.

Noninfectious conjunctivitis has been documented before in research colonies where rabbits developed severe, chronic, and purulent conjunctivitis. Microbiological testing failed to identify a causative agent for the clinical signs, and treatment with topical neomycin and hydrocortisone failed to improve discomfort and irritation. It was only when hay was moved from an overhead rack to a bundle on the floor of the cage, thereby reducing the amount of atmospheric hay dust, that the rabbits improved.[27] Keeping this laboratory case example in mind, it is important to investigate any husbandry problems that might be contributing to ocular irritation in patients. Bedding and hay should be examined for quality in cases of conjunctivitis, as well as how the hay is offered.[28]

Most cases of bacterial conjunctivitis were historically thought to be due to infections with *Pasteurella multocida*.[29] More recent studies have revealed a greater number of potential causative organisms. To interpret microbiological testing results in cases of conjunctivitis, it is important to understand the normal conjunctival flora of the rabbit. A study by Cooper and colleagues[30] in 2001 investigated the normal flora of 70 healthy domestic rabbits. They found deoxyribonuclease-negative *Staphylococcus* species to be the most frequently cultured bacteria, followed by *Micrococcus* species and *Bacillus* species. A few rabbits also grew *Stomatococcus*, *Neisseria* spp, *Pasteurella* spp, *Corynebacterium* spp, *Streptococcus* spp, and *Moraxella* spp.[30] Note that *Pasteurella*, previously thought to be the main causative agent of bacterial conjunctivitis, was found in the flora of clinically normal rabbits. And although *Staphylococcus* spp is considered a normal commensal organism, there are reports of this organism causing clinical disease.[31] Therefore, whenever any bacteria are found on culture or cytology, it is important to interpret results in light of clinical findings. Furthermore, when commensal organisms are thought to contribute to disease, it is important to look for breaches in normal host defenses, which may set up for opportunistic infection such as mechanical irritation (trichiasis, foreign body, entropion), tear film deficiencies, and or immunodeficiency.

Treatment of conjunctivitis should be aimed at addressing the underlying cause. If bacteria are thought to be the underlying cause of infection, appropriate antimicrobial therapy should be selected based on sensitivity. In cases of *Pasteurella* infection, topical chloramphenicol, ciprofloxacin, and or gentamicin 4 times daily combined with systemic broad spectrum antibiotic therapy (enrofloxacin, 10 mg/kg, twice daily) has been successful.[5] Autogenous vaccines have been used in the past for treatment of Staphylococcal conjunctivitis with initial success; however, permanent resolution was not achieved until appropriate antibiotic therapy was instituted.[32]

Viral causes of conjunctivitis must also be considered when approaching rabbits with clinical disease. Specifically, myxoma virus is known to cause inflammatory and edematous lesions of the eyelids and conjunctiva. The acute form will often lead to death before ocular signs can occur, or conjunctival hyperemia may be the only sign before death.[1,4,33] With the subacute form, conjunctival hyperemia will progress to chemosis with copious ocular exudate. Edematous and often exudative lesions around face and anogenital area are pathognomonic for the disease. Furthermore, cases of myxomatosis involve profound immunosuppression and often subsequent multifocal infection with commensal organisms[33] such as *Pasteurella*, *Pseudomonas*, and/or *Staphylococcus*. Virus isolation can be accomplished 5 days postinfection and the diagnosis made based on clinical signs and the characteristic finding of intracytoplasmic inclusion bodies in mucosal scrapings or histopathologic samples.[34] Specific treatment is not available and the prognosis is poor.[5]

CONJUNCTIVAL OVERGROWTH

Conjunctival overgrowth has been described by many names, including ankyloblepharon, pseudopterygium, conjunctival stricture, epicorneal membranous occlusion, circumferential epicorneal membranous occlusion, and or conjunctival centripetalization.[1,3,35,36] The syndrome is unique to rabbits and involves growth of a fold of conjunctival tissue arising from the limbus of the eye and extending 360° toward the axial cornea (**Fig. 6**). Unlike pterygium in humans, this conjunctival fold is nonadherent to the peripheral cornea and may appear as a narrow annulus or an extensive sheet that covers nearly the entire corneal surface.[37] The syndrome is nonpainful but can be difficult to correct, because surgical removal of the aberrant tissue is not definitive and regrowth will occur within a matter of weeks to months. Histopathology of the aberrant tissue reveals normal conjunctival epithelium and focal excess of conjunctival collagen. The condition seems to be overrepresented in young male dwarf rabbits.[22]

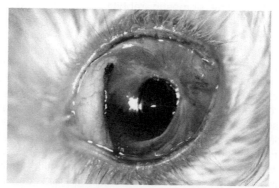

Fig. 6. Conjunctival overgrowth. (*Courtesy of* John Sapienza, DVM, DACVO; Plainview NY.)

A surgical technique has been described, which involves making centrifugal cuts into the conjunctival fold up to the limbus and lid margin. A horizontal mattress suture of 7-0 polypropylene is then made by passing the needle through the eyelid transpalpebrally and through the central rim of the conjunctival fold to manually retract the fold. Rabbits should then be treated with topical steroid ointment and the sutures left in place until they drop out. When using this method, no reoccurrence was noted in patients for 5 to 72 months of follow-up time.[35]

An alternative surgical technique was performed on a 10-month old dwarf rabbit who failed the abovementioned procedure 3 weeks postoperatively. This technique involved resecting the conjunctival membrane to the limbus and then inverting the cut edges to just behind the limbus using a Lambert suture of 6-0 polyglactin 910. The rabbit was treated with topical steroid and cyclosporine following surgery and no evidence of recurrence was noted during the follow-up period.[36]

KERATITIS

The rabbit is prone to several diseases of the corneal surface; however, traumatic injury is thought to be the most common cause.[3] Trauma can be the result of irritants from bedding or hay particles or fighting with other animals. Rabbits can also develop ulcers from underlying conditions such as entropion, distichiasis, or trichiasis. Such causes for ulceration should be investigated and treated appropriately with surgery.[3] Exposure keratitis can occur following anesthesia, with facial nerve paralysis, or with severe retrobulbar disease leading to exophthalmos and an inability to blink. Conditions such as persistent blepharitis and dacryocystitis can also lead to corneal ulceration, although these ulcers are typically ventral in location and superficial (**Fig. 7**).[1]

Superficial corneal ulceration can be managed with topical antimicrobial agents (neomycin-bacitracin-polymyxin B ophthalmic ointment 4 times daily) and topical cycloplegic medications to address painful ciliary muscle spasm and miosis.[5] With the latter, it is important to remember that rabbits have endogenous atropinase, which will affect the potency of cycloplegic medications. As with management of corneal ulceration in other species, cytology and culture can be useful in identifying concurrent microbial infection and help to recommend targeted therapy, especially if keratomalacia is present (**Fig. 8**). Although rare, there has been a report of keratomycosis in a pet rabbit.[38] After culturing *Aspergillus fumigatus*, the infection was successfully treated with topical terbinafine ointment.

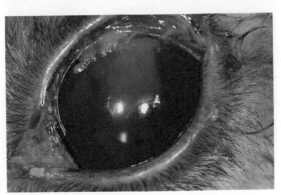

Fig. 7. Superficial corneal ulceration with concurrent conjunctivitis. (*Courtesy of* John Sapienza, DVM, DACVO; Plainview NY.)

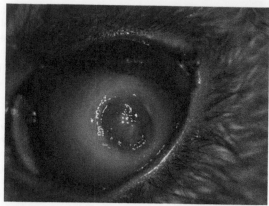

Fig. 8. Deep melting corneal ulcer. (*Courtesy of* Gerlinde Janssens, DVM; Hemiksem, Belgium)

Rabbits can also develop indolent ulcers, such as those seen in boxer dogs and corgis, with a characteristic nonadherent epithelial lip. Similarly, treatment of these ulcers requires debridement. Should simple debridement with a cotton-tipped applicator fail to produce resolution, further treatment with a grid keratotomy or anterior stromal puncture can be performed.[39,40] Placement of bandage contact lenses has also been shown to be effective in management of this disease by improving comfort level and encouraging healing.[3]

Although ulcerative keratitis is a commonly encountered problem in the rabbit, they are also known to develop noninfectious keratopathies. Distinguishing these conditions from infectious, nonulcerative keratitis has important prognosis and treatment considerations (**Fig. 9**). Lipid keratopathy is an infrequent condition that has mainly been reported in research conditions and manifests as multifocal to coalescing white refractile opacities within the cornea (**Fig. 10**). This

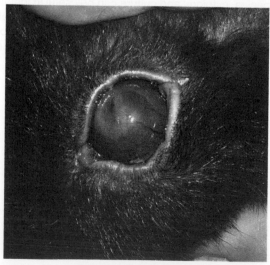

Fig. 9. Chronic keratitis with corneal scarring. (*Courtesy of* Stacy Peterson, DVM, DACVO; Albuquerque NM.)

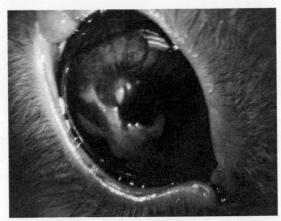

Fig. 10. Corneal lipid keratopathy. (*Courtesy of* Sinisa Grozdanic, DVM, PhD, DACVO; Hiawatha IA.)

condition has been reported in rabbits fed cholesterol-rich diets[41,42] and in rabbits fed a 10% fishmeal maintenance diet.[43] Outside of the realm of research, a case of lipid keratopathy was reported in a pet rabbit fed a predominately milk-based diet.[44] Whatever the underlying dietary cause, these lipid deposits are thought to be the result of increased uptake of low-density lipoproteins and cholesterol esters within the stromal keratocytes. These keratocytes become overwhelmed with the amount of intracellular lipid, resulting in cell death and causing the lipid and proteinaceous debris to become liberated into the corneal stroma. This debris is then phagocytosed by macrophages.[45] This process occurs in Watanabe rabbits with heritable hyperlipidemia, which have an inherited deficiency of low-density lipoprotein receptors.[41,46] Correction of the diet can help to alleviate or decrease progression of disease, and superficial keratectomy can be used to remove affected corneal tissue if extensive and visually impairing. This condition is otherwise nonpainful and often not significantly visually impairing if mild.

Corneal dystrophy has also been reported in the rabbit. Two distinct conditions have been described. The first condition appears as a unilateral, raised opaque peripheral membrane. Histologically, this condition involves areas of epithelial thinning adjacent to areas of epithelial cell hyperplasia.[47] With the other form, rabbits will have unilateral or bilateral focal, linear, or curvilinear opacities within the superficial layers of the cornea. This particular form has been seen in the American Dutch belted rabbit.[48] The underlying cause of these dystrophies has not been elucidated, but they do not seem to be painful and only become problematic if severe enough to become visually impairing.

Inflammatory keratitis has been reported in rabbits as well. Eosinophilic keratitis has been described in 2 rabbits and, similar to this disease in horses and cats, appeared as a raised, white to yellow plaque involving both the bulbar and palpebral conjunctiva, as well as the corneal surface.[49] Marked granulation tissue was present on the corneal surface, and cytology identified numerous clusters of polymorphonuclear cells with obvious intracytoplasmic eosinophilic granules. Treatment with topical neomycin-polymyxin B-dexamethasone solution 4 times daily affected resolution of clinical disease; cyclosporine treatment did not seem to be effective in managing disease long term.

SUMMARY

In summary, the domestic rabbit is prone to many of the same ocular surface diseases commonly encountered in our canine and feline domestic species, with a few exceptions. Care should always be taken to obtain a thorough history of the rabbit environment and diet at home, to determine any possible association with ocular pathology. Additionally, a complete oral examination should be performed in any case of unexplained, persistent ocular discharge and periocular inflammation. Ulcers are a frequently encountered problem in the rabbit and treatment is very similar to that of ulcers in canine patients. Provided the general practioner is familiar with a few nuances of treatment and anatomical considerations, success in treating ocular disease in the rabbit is fairly straight forward and achievable.

REFERENCES

1. Williams DL. The rabbit eye. Ophthalmology of exotic pets. Chichester (England): Wiley-Blackwell; 2012. p. 15–52.
2. Chen M, Gong L, Xu J, et al. Ultrastructural and in vivo confocal microscopic evaluation of interface after Descemet's Stripping Endothelial Keratoplasty in rabbits. Acta Ophthalmol 2012;90(1):e43–7.
3. Andrew SE. Corneal diseases of rabbits. Veterinary Clin North Am Exot Anim Pract 2002;5(2):341–56.
4. Williams DL. The rabbit. In: Gelatt KN, Gilger BC, Kern TJ, editors. Veterinary ophthalmology, vol. 2, 5th edition. Ames (IA): John Wiley & Sons, Inc.; 2013. p. 1725–49.
5. Kern TJ. Rabbit and rodent ophthalmology. Semin Avian Exot Pet Med 1997;6(3): 138–45.
6. DiGiacomo RF, Lukehart SA, Talburt CD, et al. Chronicity of infection with Treponema paraluis-cuniculi in New Zealand white rabbits. Genitourin Med 1985;61(3): 156–64.
7. DiGiacomo RF, Lukehart SA, Talburt CD, et al. Clinical course and treatment of venereal spirochaetosis in New Zealand white rabbits. Br J Vener Dis 1984; 60(4):214–8.
8. Burling K, Murphy CH, Curiel JS. Anatomy of the rabbits nasolacrimal duct and its clinical implications. Prog Vet Comp Ophthalmol 1991;1:33–40.
9. Mullan SM, Main DC. Survey of the husbandry, health and welfare of 102 pet rabbits. Vet Rec 2006;159(4):103–9.
10. Florin M, Rusanen E, Haessig M, et al. Clinical presentation, treatment, and outcome of dacryocystitis in rabbits: a retrospective study of 28 cases (2003-2007). Vet Ophthalmol 2009;12(6):350–6.
11. Brown C. Nasolacrimal duct lavage in rabbits. Lab Anim (NY) 2006;35(6):22–4.
12. Marini RP, Foltz CJ, Kersten D, et al. Microbiologic, radiographic, and anatomic study of the nasolacrimal duct apparatus in the rabbit (Oryctolagus cuniculus). Lab Anim Sci 1996;46(6):656–62.
13. Goldstein SM, Katowitz JA, Syed NA. The histopathologic effects of balloon dacryoplasty on the rabbit nasolacrimal duct. J AAPOS 2006;10(4):333–5.
14. Sakai T. Major ocular glands (harderian gland and lacrimal gland) of the musk shrew (Suncus murinus) with a review on the comparative anatomy and histology of the mammalian lacrimal glands. J Morphol 1989;201(1):39–57.
15. Maurice D. The effect of the low blink rate in rabbits on topical drug penetration. J Ocul Pharmacol Ther 1995;11(3):297–304.

16. Gilbard JP, Dartt DA. Changes in rabbit lacrimal gland fluid osmolarity with flow rate. Invest Ophthalmol Vis Sci 1982;23(6):804–6.
17. Trousdale MD, Zhu Z, Stevenson D, et al. Expression of TNF inhibitor gene in the lacrimal gland promotes recovery of tear production and tear stability and reduced immunopathology in rabbits with induced autoimmune dacryoadenitis. J Autoimmune Dis 2005;2:6.
18. Lima L, Lange RR, Turner-Giannico A, et al. Evaluation of standardized endodontic paper point tear test in New Zealand white rabbits and comparison between corneal sensitivity followed tear tests. Vet Ophthalmol 2015;18(Suppl 1):119–24.
19. Whittaker AL, Williams DL. Evaluation of lacrimation characteristics in clinically normal New Zealand White Rabbits by Using the Schirmer Tear Test I. J Am Assoc Lab Anim Sci 2015;54(6):783–7.
20. Biricik HS, Oguz H, Sindak N, et al. Evaluation of the Schirmer and phenol red thread tests for measuring tear secretion in rabbits. Vet Rec 2005;156(15):485–7.
21. Hamano H, Hori M, Hamano T, et al. A new method for measuring tears. CLAO J 1983;9(3):281–9.
22. Abrams KL, Brooks DE, Funk RS, et al. Evaluation of the Schirmer tear test in clinically normal rabbits. Am J Vet Res 1990;51(12):1912–3.
23. Thomas PB, Zhu Z, Selvam S, et al. Autoimmune dacryoadenitis and keratoconjunctivitis induced in rabbits by subcutaneous injection of autologous lymphocytes activated ex vivo against lacrimal antigens. J Autoimmun 2008;31(2):116–22.
24. Nagelhout TJ, Gamache DA, Roberts L, et al. Preservation of tear film integrity and inhibition of corneal injury by dexamethasone in a rabbit model of lacrimal gland inflammation-induced dry eye. J Ocul Pharmacol Ther 2005;21(2):139–48.
25. Thomas PB, Samant DM, Zhu Z, et al. Long-term topical cyclosporine treatment improves tear production and reduces keratoconjunctivitis in rabbits with induced autoimmune dacryoadenitis. J Ocul Pharmacol Ther 2009;25(3):285–92.
26. Shirani D, Selk Ghaffari M, Akbarein H, et al. Effects of short-term oral administration of trimethoprim-sulfamethoxazole on Schirmer II tear test results in clinically normal rabbits. Vet Rec 2010;166(20):623–4.
27. Buckley P, Lowman DM. Chronic non-infective conjunctivitis in rabbits. Lab Anim 1979;13(2):69–73.
28. McGary ED, Young BE. Quantitative determination of zinc, iron, calcium, and phosphorus in the total diet market basket by atomic absorption and colorimetric spectrophotometry. J Agric Food Chem 1976;24(3):539–42.
29. Okerman L, Devriese LA, Maertens L, et al. Cutaneous staphylococcosis in rabbits. Vet Rec 1984;114(13):313–5.
30. Cooper SC, McLellan GJ, Rycroft AN. Conjunctival flora observed in 70 healthy domestic rabbits (Oryctolagus cuniculus). Vet Rec 2001;149(8):232–5.
31. Snyder SB, Fox JG, Campbell LH, et al. Disseminated staphylococcal disease in laboratory rabbits (Oryctolagus cuniculus). Lab Anim Sci 1976;26(1):86–8.
32. Hinton M. Treatment of purulent staphylococcal conjunctivitis in rabbits with autogenous vaccine. Lab Anim 1977;11(3):163–4.
33. Fenner F, Woodroofe GM. The pathogenesis of infectious myxomatosis; the mechanism of infection and the immunological response in the European rabbit (Oryctolagus cuniculus). Br J Exp Pathol 1953;34(4):400–11.
34. Patton NM, Holmes HT. Myxomatosis in domestic rabbits in Oregon. J Am Vet Med Assoc 1977;171(6):560–2.
35. Allgower I, Malho P, Shulze H, Schaffer E. Aberrant conjunctival stricture and overgrowth in the rabbit. Vet Ophthalmol 2008;11(1):18–22.

36. Kim JY, Williams DL, Rho KS, et al. Surgical correction of aberrant conjunctival overgrowth in a rabbit: a case report. Ir Vet J 2013;66(1):18.
37. Roze M, Ridings B, Lagadic M. Comparative morphology of epicorneal conjunctival membranes in rabbits and human pterygium. Vet Ophthalmol 2001;4(3):171–4.
38. Bourguet A, Guyonnet A, Donzel E, et al. Keratomycosis in a pet rabbit (Oryctolagus cuniculus) treated with topical 1% terbinafine ointment. Vet Ophthalmol 2016;19(6):504–9.
39. Bentley E, Abrams GA, Covitz D, et al. Morphology and immunohistochemistry of spontaneous chronic corneal epithelial defects (SCCED) in dogs. Invest Ophthalmol Vis Sci 2001;42(10):2262–9.
40. Murphy CJ, Marfurt CF, McDermott A, et al. Spontaneous chronic corneal epithelial defects (SCCED) in dogs: clinical features, innervation, and effect of topical SP, with or without IGF-1. Invest Ophthalmol Vis Sci 2001;42(10):2252–61.
41. Kouchi M, Ueda Y, Horie H, et al. Ocular lesions in Watanabe heritable hyperlipidemic rabbits. Vet Ophthalmol 2006;9(3):145–8.
42. Fallon MT, Reinhard MK, DaRif CA, et al. Diagnostic exercise: eye lesions in a rabbit. Lab Anim Sci 1988;38(5):612–3.
43. Sebesteny A, Sheraidah GA, Trevan DJ, et al. Lipid keratopathy and atheromatosis in an SPF laboratory rabbit colony attributable to diet. Lab Anim 1985;19(3):180–8.
44. Gwin RM, Gelatt KN. Bilateral ocular lipidosis in a cottontail rabbit fed an all-milk diet. J Am Vet Med Assoc 1977;171(9):887–9.
45. Roth SI, Stock EL, Siel JM, et al. Pathogenesis of experimental lipid keratopathy. An ultrastructural study of an animal model system. Invest Ophthalmol Vis Sci 1988;29(10):1544–51.
46. Garibaldi BA, Goad ME. Lipid keratopathy in the Watanabe (WHHL) rabbit. Vet Pathol 1988;25(2):173–4.
47. Port CD, Dodd DC. Two cases of corneal epithelial dystrophy in rabbits. Lab Anim Sci 1983;33(6):587–8.
48. Moore CP, Dubielzig R, Glaza SM. Anterior corneal dystrophy of American Dutch belted rabbits: biomicroscopic and histopathologic findings. Vet Pathol 1987;24(1):28–33.
49. Grinninger P, Sanchez R, Kraijer-Huver IM, et al. Eosinophilic keratoconjunctivitis in two rabbits. Vet Ophthalmol 2012;15(1):59–65.

Ocular Surface Disease in Rodents (Guinea Pigs, Mice, Rats, Chinchillas)

Caroline Monk, DVM, DACVO

KEYWORDS

- Cornea • Chromodacryorrhea • Dystrophy • Conjunctivitis • Scurvy
- Keratoconjunctivitis sicca

KEY POINTS

- The small size of rodent eyes makes examination and individualized treatment challenging.
- As with all exotic species, improper husbandry plays a disproportionate role in the development of many rodent corneal diseases.
- Although rodent eyes have their own unique anatomy, they remain susceptible to many of the same diseases that affect dogs and cats. Emphasis has been placed on conditions unique to the species discussed herein.
- Mice and rats frequently present with varying forms of corneal opacification and deposits that may not be of clinical significance.
- Rodents are hypsodonts, with enamel extending past the gum line and a continuous growth of their teeth, making them highly susceptible to uneven wear and overgrowth that can be reflected in secondary ocular disease.

INTRODUCTION

Rodents are mammals of the order *Rodentia*, and constitute up to 40% of all known mammal species. Rodents are defined by their hypsodont dentition, with continuously growing incisors of the upper and lower jaw. The species discussed herein are domesticated from their wild counterparts for laboratory, farm, and pet purposes. The presence of inbred strains, most notably in mice and rats, must be considered when examining pet rodents, as many originate from laboratory strains. These genetic ocular defects are occasionally sought as models for human disease, but they can also be unwelcome byproducts linked to the desired trait. As social species that naturally live in colonies, herd management and individual welfare may be presented to the

The author has nothing to disclose.
Ophthalmology, BluePearl Veterinary Partners, 1071 Howell Mill Road Northwest, Atlanta, GA 30318, USA
E-mail address: caroline.monk@bluepearlvet.com

attending veterinarian. Mice, rats, and chinchillas are thought to be predominantly nocturnal to crepuscular, while guinea pigs are diurnal. Their eye anatomy reflects their origins. All rodents have a cornea divided into stratified epithelium, a Bowman layer (epithelial basement membrane), stroma, Descemet membrane, and the endothelium.

GUINEA PIG (*CAVIA PORCELLUS*)

Guinea pigs are the largest of the rodents covered in this section. They live an average of 4 to 5 years, but can live as long as 8 years. They are not found in the wild, but are a domesticated relative of other species of cavies. Once used frequently for research studies, they are now primarily a household pet.

Normal Anatomy

Fine superficial corneal neovascularization (usually extending from limbus axially to the first or second third of the cornea) has been reported as a normal finding in fetal, newborn, and adult guinea pigs.[1] However, a later confocal microscopy study did not confirm this.[2]

Small palpebral conjunctival outpouchings were noted in the upper and lower fornices in almost all examined animals according to Dwyer and colleagues (1983), and were determined via histology to be masses of lymphoid tissue. Their prevalence across individuals resulted in researchers concluding these foci to be a normal finding.

Guinea pigs have a remarkably low corneal sensitivity (or a high pressure threshold is needed to elicit a blink), replicated in 3 studies.[1,3,4] In these studies, the guinea pig was observed to have limited to no reflex tearing, which may be a component of the lack of corneal sensitivity (**Fig. 1**, **Table 1**). This plays an important clinical role.

Staphylococcus epidermidis, α-hemolytic *Streptococcus*, and *Corynebacterium* were the top 3 aerobic commensal isolates from normal healthy guinea pigs.[4]

Adnexa-Related Corneal Disease

Trichiasis, or hair from the skin contacting the cornea, occurs in a wire-haired breed of guinea pigs, Texel cavies; 0.8% of surveyed animals had this congenital abnormality.[11] After birth the wiry hair can curl inwards into the eye, causing corneal ulcers and epiphora. Lubricating the eyes and hair around frequently immediately after birth until the hair grows in a more controlled manner can help.

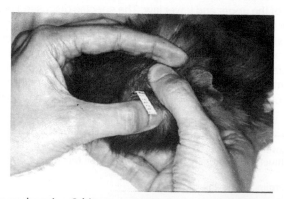

Fig. 1. Guinea pig undergoing Schirmer tear test. Guinea pigs have been shown to have a remarkably insensitive cornea relative to other domesticated species, and little to no reflex tearing. (*Courtesy of* Dr Stacy Andrew.)

Table 1
Corneal parameter

	STT 1 (mm/min)	PRTT (mm/15 s)	CTT (g/mm^2)
Guinea pig	3 mm[4]	21.2 ± 4.2[4]	6.64[4]
	0.36 ± 1.1 (Duncan Hartley cavies)[5]	16.0 ± 4.7[5]	3.7[5]
	9.65 ± 3.5 (used a 3 × 35 mm strip instead of traditional 5 × 40 mm)[3]		7.75[3]
Mouse & Rat		6 – 8[6]	~0.96 (6 cm)[7]
			~12.8 (0.8 ± 0.9 mm, sedated rats, author noted result was unusually high)[8]
Chinchilla	1.07 ± 0.54[9]	14.6 ± 3.5[10]	~10.84 (1.24 ± 0.46 cm)[9]
			1.5 ± 0.9[10]

Selected tear film parameters in rodents. Mean ± standard deviation is included when available. Corneal sensitivity is reported in g/mm^2. When applicable, a standard conversion table for Cochet-Bonnet aesthesiometer was used to convert from cm to g/mm^2. Range: 6.0-0.5 cm = 0.96-17.68 g/mm^2.

Entropion, either primary or cicatrial after an eyelid trauma, is reported in guinea pigs. Entropion is typically treated via a variety of blepharoplasties. To the author's knowledge, blepharoplasty in a guinea pig has not been reported. Because of their small adnexal structures, they may be more suited to a hyaluronate injection that can evert the lids semipermanently or to frequent lubrication of the cornea to mitigate pathology.

Primary Corneal Disease

To the author's knowledge, guinea pigs are the only species discussed in this article formally reported to exhibit periocular dermoids.[12] Large corneal dermoids can compromise vision by their opacification of the visual axis. Haired dermoids may contaminate the conjunctival sac by harboring foreign material and debris. The treatment of choice for dermoids is surgical removal via keratectomy, but given the thinness of the guinea pig cornea (**Table 2**), this treatment should be undertaken with great care.

Table 2
Selected corneal parameters in rodents and their respective method of measurement. Mean ± standard deviation is included when available

	Central Corneal Thickness (μm)	Endothelial Cell Count (Peak, Cells/mm^2)	Mechanism of Measurement (Respectively)
Guinea pig	227.85 ± 14.09[2]	2352 ± 49[2]	Pachymetry Confocal
Mouse	108.0 ± 5.1[13] 106.0 ± 3.45[14]	1587 ± 74[15]	Optical coherence tomography Optical low coherence reflectometer Confocal
Rat	159.08 ± 14.99 (Winstar)[14]	1951 ± 67[15] 3744 (Lewis)[16]	Optical low coherence reflectometer Confocal Histology
Chinchilla	340 ± 30[9]	3423[17]	Pachymetry Contact specular microscope

Corneal lipidosis (bilateral stromal lipid dystrophy) is also reported.[11] This has been described as a bilateral paracentral lipid deposition with varying degrees of density and coverage. This appears to be less common than the corneal dystrophy reported in mice and rats.

Corneal Foreign Bodies

As previously discussed, guinea pigs have been found to have a low corneal sensitivity and a negligible ability to produce reflex tears, thereby placing them at an unusual risk for ocular foreign bodies. They have also been noted to have an unusually low blink rate.[2,5] This is compounded by their typical housing, in a bedded enclosure with straw and hay at eye level. In a survey of 1000 guinea pigs, 4.7% had conjunctivitis, which was frequently secondary to a traumatic injury from a foreign body.[11] This had also been seen in a previous survey of guinea pigs.[1] It has been theorized that the corneal vessels and lymphoid tissue unique to guinea pigs eyes were an evolved strategy over increased blinking and discomfort seen in other animals. That being said, foreign bodies should still be taken seriously and treated promptly. Per Williams and Sullivan (2010), these foreign bodies, along with congenital trichiasis, seemed to be the most irritating for the animals.

Treatment Considerations

Guinea pigs have lost their ability to endogenously form ascorbic acid, like people and capybaras, and are therefore at greater risk for scurvy relative to other species of rodent. Scurvy often starts with mucous membrane disease including petechiation and ulceration. Dry eye has also been reported as a sequela. Vitamin C is used in other species as an anticollagenase.[18] Therefore, supplementation during times of ulceration, especially a melting ulcer (**Fig. 2**), is likely to be beneficial regardless of nutritional status. Many foods are rich in vitamin C, and there are also nutritional supplements available.

Because guinea pigs are the largest of the species discussed here, topical treatment is more feasible in terms of administration. Systemic absorption is still a risk, and so prolonged treatment, especially with topical steroids and nonsteroidal anti-inflammatory drugs, should be approached cautiously. Guinea pigs are typically docile and amenable to handling. Given their common place as a household pet, individualized treatment including frequent topical medication is more achievable.

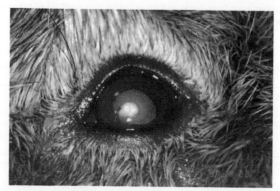

Fig. 2. Infected corneal ulcer in a guinea pig. This is a disease process in which guinea pigs would benefit from additional supplementation of vitamin C for normal physiology and also for its anticollagenolytic properties. (*Courtesy of* Dr Stacy Andrew.)

MICE (*MUS*)

Mice are the smallest rodent discussed in this section. They are one of the most successful mammals on Earth today and are viewed as pets, research subjects, vermin, and vectors. They are the most common experimental laboratory animal in recent decades because of their homology with people, small size, and rapid reproduction. Breeding onset is about 50 days, and the life span is typically 1 to 2 years when kept as pet.

Normal Anatomy

A detailed comparative study was performed using confocal microscopy of normal 4-month-old Swiss mice.[15] Bowman layer was observed between basal epithelial cells and the anterior stroma. Similar to rats, the anterior and posterior stroma had numerous anuclear reflective stellate structures. Endothelial cell density was also determined (see **Table 2**).

Just like guinea pigs, corneal vascularization has been reported to be a normal finding in 2 mouse strains – athymic and euthymic nude mice.[19]

Schirmer tear test with traditional Whatman filter paper is not possible in the species based on size, but normal tear volume can be assessed via phenol red thread testing (see **Table 1**).[6]

Mice in Research

No article on mice would be complete without touching on their significance as a research model.

Mice are models for certain ocular surface diseases, most notably Sjögren syndrome (SS), a common autoimmune dry eye syndrome in people. Mice exhibiting SS-like characteristics have a mononuclear cell infiltration into exocrine glands, loss of acinar tissue, and secretory dysfunction. Corneal pathology includes corneal vascularization, keratinization, and the propensity for bacterial corneal ulcers (**Fig. 3**). Numerous murine strains have been used for their SS-like disease manifestations,

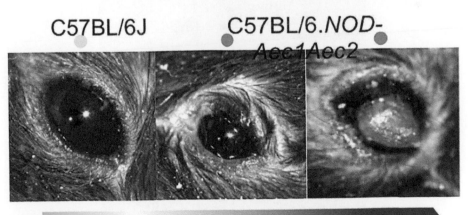

Fig. 3. Ocular pathology associated with mouse models of Sjögren syndrome. Here one can see disease ranging from a clear corneal with mild discharge, to blepharospasm and keratitis, all the way to a stromal corneal ulcer with secondary infection. (*Courtesy of* Dr Renata Ramos.)

and an excellent review article summarizing the various models has been published.[20] Initially these characteristics were spontaneously arising, but later the alterations were associated with gene knockout, resulting in transgenic mice that model aspects of the disease.

Mice have helped make a breakthrough in the link between primary open-angle glaucoma and the thickness of the central cornea. Mice were recently used to identify a transcription factor, POU6F2, that is associated with central corneal thickness and susceptibility of retinal ganglion cells to injury.[21]

Primary Corneal Disease

Corneal deposits are a common finding in laboratory mice (**Fig. 4**). Deposition of calcium in Bowman layer with or without accompanying vascularization has been reported in both normal and SS-model mice (MRL/Mp strain).[22] It is speculated that these deposits are genetically linked, but excess ammonia in cage bedding may also contribute.[23] After investigating husbandry, treatment of the deposits is not performed.

Peter anomaly, a form of anterior segment dysgenesis, has been documented spontaneously mice and is being used as a model for the disease.[24,25] The keratolenticular adhesion results in the presence of a leukoma (corneal opacity) of varying size. Corneal transplant is the treatment in people, but even then overall visual prognosis is poor.[26] This treatment has not been reported in veterinary patients. Additionally, intraocular pressure should be assessed, as aggressive glaucoma often accompanies these changes.[24]

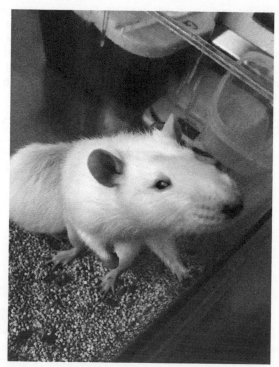

Fig. 4. Severe example of corneal dystrophy in a laboratory mouse. This individual was considered comfortable (no blepharospasm) and clinically acceptable as a research subject.

Treatment Considerations

The primary limiting factor in treatment of mice is their small size. Corneal transplants have been performed successfully, but the success rate of these surgeries has not been published, as most studies focus on graft rejection, excluding those leaking or infected grafts from statistical analysis.[27,28] In veterinary medicine, conjunctival grafts are more commonly performed relative to clear corneal transplants, but to the author's knowledge, this surgical technique has not been reported in any the species covered in this article.

The small size of the mouse also means many topical treatments have the potential for significant systemic absorption. Even the application of a topical sodium channel blocker to facilitate examination should be applied with judiciousness given its potential for systemic toxicity.[29]

RATS (*RATTUS*)

Rats and mice are closely related and only differentiated by their size, not specific taxonomic criteria. This section focuses on the most common rat species, *Rattus norvegicus* (brown rat and laboratory rat), *Rattus rattus* (black rat), and fancy rat (*Rattus norvegicus*). Life span is typically 2 years when kept as a pet, but they can live up to 3 years.

Normal Anatomy

Rats and mice have 3 tear-producing glands, the intraorbital, the extraorbital, and the Harderian. The Harderian is a well-studied exocrine gland associated with the third eyelid. This is what produces the porphyrin and lipid-laden tears in rats and is of clinical significance because of the vivid, visible tears it produces in several diseases.[30]

Adnexa-Related Corneal Disease

Tear staining or chromodacryorrhea refers to a dark stain below the inner corner of the eye, caused by porphyrin-pigmented secretion from the Harderian gland. It indicates stress in rats but can have other indirect causes. Chromodacryorrhea was produced within 15 minutes in young rats following intravenous injection of acetylcholine or acute stress induced by limb restraint.[31] By a similar mechanism, the presence of chromodacryorrhea was even identified as a welfare indicator on commercial pig farms.[32] This finding may gain more attention in the laboratory animal sphere, where welfare is paramount. The presence of chromodacryorrhea should not be ignored, as it is not a normal finding. As discussed, it may be caused by environmental stress, physical illness, or underlying disease. Furthermore, even when not hypersecreted, porphyrins are labile until photic energy. Exposure to high-intensity light induced necrosis of the glandular cells in a study on a research population of Wistar rats.[33] The injury appeared to be caused by the creation of free radicals within glandular cells, probably as a result of photodynamic action on the porphyrins in the gland. Proper husbandry with a day-night cycle is essential for rat health and welfare.

Primary Corneal Disease

Certain strains of rat are reported to have a high rate of subepithelial mineralization (corneal dystrophy), just like mice. Clinically, these opacities are subepithelial (associated with abnormal epithelial basement membrane, Bowman layer). They vary from a few punctate opacities only visible with a slit lamp to marked dense opacities covering a majority of the corneal surface (**Fig. 5**). A thorough ophthalmologic and histopathological study was performed on Fischer-344 (F344) rats that demonstrated a high incidence of corneal basement membrane dystrophy.[34] In the most severely affected

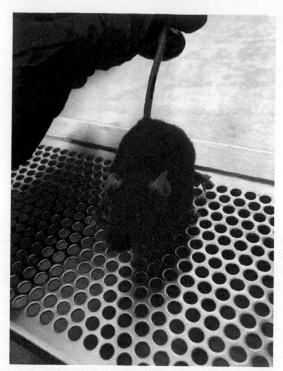

Fig. 5. Another example of severe corneal dystrophy, this time in a laboratory rat. Just like the mouse example, no blepharospasm was exhibited by this individual.

strains, this correlated to a systemic basement membrane disorder. It was speculated that these opacities are relatively under-reported for several reasons, and in this study anywhere from 50% to 100% of rats examined from various breeders had corneal dystrophy. Thankfully, these opacifications did not appear to cause the animals discomfort or have an adverse effect on normal physiologic function. However, in people, epithelial basement membrane dystrophy is associated with recurrent corneal erosions.[35]

F344 rat strains are also unusually prone to intraocular tumor, which may manifest as a pigmented opacity in the cornea. Orbital malignant schwannomas and amelanotic melanoma are reported.[36]

Infectious Corneal Disease

Sialodacryoadenitis (SDA) is a highly contagious common viral infection in rats. SDA is caused by rat coronavirus and can spread rapidly, especially through laboratory colonies. Anorexia occurs during these viral infections. The virus has a tropism for epithelial cells and can infect the Harderian and extraorbital glands, causing ocular disease.[37] Often, lacrimal gland involvement leads to reduced tear production. Young rats are especially susceptible to SDA, and the infection can occur in the lower respiratory tract, resulting in pneumonia. Thankfully, the primary disease is usually self-limiting and resolves within a week; however, secondary signs may take up to a month to fully resolve. Diagnosis is confirmed by detecting coronavirus antigen with reverse transcriptase polymerase chain reaction (RT-PCR)[38] or serologic testing.[39]

Treatment Considerations

Treatment limitations are similar between rats and mice. Their small size and colony habitat often preclude topical treatment.

CHINCHILLA (DOMESTICATED FROM *CHINCHILLA LANIGERA*)

Of the species covered, chinchillas are the most recently domesticated and the least studied. They are also the longest lived in this group of rodents, living on average 10 years in captivity, although chinchillas living into their 20s have been reported.[10] Chinchillas were originally bred for fur but since have become pets and are used in scientific research. Of the species discussed here, chinchillas have the most recent literature regarding presentation as a pet for ocular examination, and less research-based publications relating to their ocular biology. In a recent retrospective study over the course of 10 years, 7.8% of chinchillas presenting to a tertiary clinic had primary ophthalmic complaints.[10]

Normal Anatomy

Chinchillas are characterized as having a shallow orbit, and proptosis can easily be induced with pressure on the eyelids; therefore, care must be taken when examining them.[40] Chinchilla endothelial cell density has been determined via specular microscopy (see **Table 2**).[17] Like in other species, cell density decreases and pleomorphism increases with age.

Adnexa-Related Corneal Disease

Of the available publications and consensus among zoo veterinarians, ocular discharge appears to be the most common condition. The discharge/epiphora is suspected to be secondary to dental disease, as in all rodents, chinchillas are hypsodonts with continually growing teeth. This continual growth is compounded by their longevity and potential for inappropriate husbandry.[41] Root extension into the nasolacrimal duct and subsequent epiphora is the most common clinical sign. Chinchillas with only clear epiphora are typically considered primary dental disease patients.[10]

Infectious Corneal Disease

Bacteria normally populate the conjunctival fornix. In chinchillas,[9] Lima and colleagues (2010) found that *Streptococcus* species (27.45%) was most commonly isolated, followed by *Staphylococcus aureus* (23.52%), and finally coagulase-negative *Staphylococcus* (19.60%). This is in comparison to[42] Ozawa and colleagues (2017), who studied chinchillas affected by bacterial conjunctivitis. In diseased individuals, 61.5% yielded a gram-negative isolate (50% being *Pseudomonas aeruginosa*). The remainder yielded gram-positive isolates, *Staphylococcus* species being most common (26.9%). Chinchillas with acute conjunctivitis (1–3 days) were much more commonly affected by gram-negative organisms, and most cases were unilateral; 36.7% had concurrent dental disease.

Treatment Considerations

As chinchillas often experience conjunctivitis secondary to other disease, a thorough dental examination addressing the underlying cause is essential. However, despite this clinical paradigm, most chinchillas with bacterial conjunctivitis are reported to fully resolved with topical with or without oral antimicrobial therapy within 3 weeks.[42] Being larger in size than rats and mice and more typically housed in a pet environment, chinchillas may be more amenable to topical medication, similar to guinea pigs.

SUMMARY

Most diseases specific to rodents are either congenital or related to husbandry. Unfortunately, their small size limits many of the typical surgical treatments routinely performed in other veterinary species. Once husbandry is addressed, treatment may be limited to mitigation of the disease process but not complete resolution.

REFERENCES

1. Dwyer RS, Darougar S, Monnickendam MA. Unusual features in the conjunctiva and cornea of the normal guinea-pig: clinical and histological studies. Br J Ophthalmol 1983;67(11):737–41.
2. Cafaro TA, Ortiz SG, Maldonado C, et al. The cornea of Guinea pig: structural and functional studies. Vet Ophthalmol 2009;12(4):234–41.
3. Wieser B, Tichy A, Nell B. Correlation between corneal sensitivity and quantity of reflex tearing in cows, horses, goats, sheep, dogs, cats, rabbits, and guinea pigs. Vet Ophthalmol 2013;16(4):251–62.
4. Coster ME, Stiles J, Krohne SG, et al. Results of diagnostic ophthalmic testing in healthy guinea pigs. J Am Vet Med Assoc 2008;232(12):1825–33.
5. Trost K, Skalicky M, Nell B. Schirmer tear test, phenol red thread tear test, eye blink frequency and corneal sensitivity in the guinea pig. Vet Ophthalmol 2007; 10(3):143–6.
6. Lin Z, Liu X, Zhou T, et al. A mouse dry eye model induced by topical administration of benzalkonium chloride. Mol Vis 2011;17:257–64.
7. Chucair-Elliott AJ, Zheng M, Carr DJJ. Degeneration and regeneration of corneal nerves in response to HSV-1 infection. Invest Ophthalmol Vis Sci 2015;56(2): 1097–107.
8. Kim J, Kim N-S, Lee K-C, et al. Effect of topical anesthesia on evaluation of corneal sensitivity and intraocular pressure in rats and dogs. Vet Ophthalmol 2013;16(1):43–6.
9. Lima L, Montiani-Ferreira F, Tramontin M, et al. The chinchilla eye: morphologic observations, echobiometric findings and reference values for selected ophthalmic diagnostic tests. Vet Ophthalmol 2010;13(Suppl):14–25.
10. Müller K, Mauler DA, Eule JC. Reference values for selected ophthalmic diagnostic tests and clinical characteristics of chinchilla eyes (Chinchilla lanigera). Vet Ophthalmol 2010;13(Suppl):29–34.
11. Williams D, Sullivan A. Ocular disease in the guinea pig (Cavia porcellus): a survey of 1000 animals. Vet Ophthalmol 2010;13(Suppl):54–62.
12. Wappler O, Allgoewer I, Schaeffer EH. Conjunctival dermoid in two guinea pigs: a case report. Vet Ophthalmol 2002;5(3):245–8.
13. Chatterjee A, Oh D-J, Kang MH, et al. Central corneal thickness does not correlate with TonoLab-Measured IOP in several mouse strains with single transgenic mutations of matricellular proteins. Exp Eye Res 2013;115:106–12.
14. Schulz D, Iliev ME, Frueh BE, et al. In vivo pachymetry in normal eyes of rats, mice and rabbits with the optical low coherence reflectometer. Vis Res 2003; 43(6):723–8.
15. Labbé A, Liang H, Martin C, et al. Comparative anatomy of laboratory animal corneas with a new-generation high-resolution in vivo confocal microscope. Curr Eye Res 2006;31(6):501–9.
16. Bredow L, Schwartzkopff J, Reinhard T. Regeneration of corneal endothelial cells following keratoplasty in rats with bullous keratopathy. Mol Vis 2014;20:683–90.

17. Bercht BS, Albuquerque L, Araujo ACP, et al. Specular microscopy to determine corneal endothelial cell morphology and morphometry in chinchillas (Chinchilla lanigera) in vivo. Vet Ophthalmol 2015;18(Suppl 1):137–42.
18. Cho Y-W, Yoo W-S, Kim S-J, et al. Efficacy of systemic vitamin C supplementation in reducing corneal opacity resulting from infectious keratitis. Medicine (Baltimore) 2014;93(23):e125.
19. Niederkorn JY, Ubelaker JE, Martin JM. Vascularization of corneas of hairless mutant mice. Invest Ophthalmol Vis Sci 1990;31(5):948–53.
20. Delaleu N, Nguyen CQ, Peck AB, et al. Sjögren's syndrome: studying the disease in mice. Arthritis Res Ther 2011;13(3):217.
21. King R, Struebing FL, Li Y, et al. Genomic locus modulating corneal thickness in the mouse identifies POU6F2 as a potential risk of developing glaucoma. PLoS Genet 2018;14(1):e1007145.
22. Verhagen C, Rowshani T, Willekens B, et al. Spontaneous development of corneal crystalline deposits in MRL/Mp mice. Invest Ophthalmol Vis Sci 1995;36(2):454–61.
23. Rosenbaum MD, VandeWoude S, Johnson TE. Effects of cage-change frequency and bedding volume on mice and their microenvironment. J Am Assoc Lab Anim Sci 2009;48(6):763–73.
24. Mao M, Kiss M, Ou Y, et al. Genetic dissection of anterior segment dysgenesis caused by a Col4a1 mutation in mouse. Dis Model Mech 2017;10(4):475–85.
25. Hägglund A-C, Jones I, Carlsson L. A novel mouse model of anterior segment dysgenesis (ASD): conditional deletion of Tsc1 disrupts ciliary body and iris development. Dis Model Mech 2017;10(3):245–57.
26. Rao KV, Fernandes M, Gangopadhyay N, et al. Outcome of penetrating keratoplasty for Peters anomaly. Cornea 2008;27(7):749–53.
27. Hori J, Streilein JW. Dynamics of donor cell persistence and recipient cell replacement in orthotopic corneal allografts in mice. Invest Ophthalmol Vis Sci 2001;42(8):1820–8.
28. Li S, Yu J, Guo C, et al. The balance of Th1/Th2 and LAP+Tregs/Th17 cells is crucial for graft survival in allogeneic corneal transplantation. J Ophthalmol 2018;2018:5404989.
29. Ohmura S, Kawada M, Ohta T, et al. Systemic toxicity and resuscitation in bupivacaine-, levobupivacaine-, or ropivacaine-infused rats. Anesth Analg 2001;93(3):743–8.
30. Walling BE, Marit GB. The eye and harderian gland [Chapter 12]. In: Parker GA, Picut CA, editors. Atlas of histology of the juvenile rat. Boston: Academic Press; 2016. p. 373–94.
31. Harkness JE, Ridgway MD. Chromodacryorrhea in laboratory rats (Rattus norvegicus): etiologic considerations. Lab Anim Sci 1980;30(5):841–4.
32. Telkänranta H, Marchant-Forde JN, Valros A. Tear staining in pigs: a potential tool for welfare assessment on commercial farms. Animal: An International Journal of Animal Bioscience 2016;10(2):318–25.
33. Kurisu K, Sawamoto O, Watanabe H, et al. Sequential changes in the Harderian gland of rats exposed to high intensity light. Lab Anim Sci 1996;46(1):71–6.
34. Bruner RH, Keller WF, Stitzel KA, et al. Spontaneous corneal dystrophy and generalized basement membrane changes in Fischer-344 rats. Toxicol Pathol 1992;20(3 Pt 1):357–66.
35. Laibson PR. Recurrent corneal erosions and epithelial basement membrane dystrophy. Eye Contact Lens 2010;36(5):315–7.

36. Yoshitomi K, Boorman GA. Intraocular and orbital malignant Schwannomas in F344 rats. Vet Pathol 1991;28(6):457–66.
37. Compton SR, Smith AL, Gaertner DJ. Comparison of the pathogenicity in rats of rat coronaviruses of different neutralization groups. Lab Anim Sci 1999;49(5): 514–8.
38. Compton SR, Vivas-Gonzalez BE, Macy JD. Reverse transcriptase polymerase chain reaction-based diagnosis and molecular characterization of a new rat coronavirus strain. Lab Anim Sci 1999;49(5):506–13.
39. Percy DH, Scott RA. Coronavirus infection in the laboratory rat: immunization trials using attenuated virus replicated in L-2 cells. Can J Vet Res 1991;55(1):60–6.
40. Peiffer RL, Johnson PT. Clinical ocular findings in a colony of chinchillas (Chinchilla laniger). Lab Anim 1980;14(4):331–5.
41. Crossley DA, Miguélez MM. Skull size and cheek-tooth length in wild-caught and captive-bred chinchillas. Arch Oral Biol 2001;46(10):919–28.
42. Ozawa S, Mans C, Szabo Z, et al. Epidemiology of bacterial conjunctivitis in chinchillas (Chinchilla lanigera): 49 cases (2005 to 2015). J Small Anim Pract 2017; 58(4):238–45.

Ocular Examination and Corneal Surface Disease in the Ferret

Kathern E. Myrna, DVM, MS, DACVO[a],*,
Nicola Di Girolamo, DMV, GPCert (ExAP), MSc (EBHC), PhD, DECZM (Herpetology)[b]

KEYWORDS

- Ferret • Ophthalmology • Cornea • Mustela • Corneal scar • Eyes

KEY POINTS

- Ocular examination of the ferret can be challenging and requires a systematic approach.
- Ferret ophthalmic disease is uncommon.
- Ferrets eyes are small and relatively well protected but they can still experience corneal surface trauma.

INTRODUCTION

Although ferrets have become popular companion animals, most knowledge on ocular diseases of the ferret comes from research into the development of the retina. This has created a paucity of reliable resources on ferret ophthalmology in clinical practice. This article reviews practical techniques for examining the domestic ferret (*Mustela putorius furo*) and reviews the most common diseases of the cornea and conjunctiva in ferrets.

OCULAR EXAMINATION

Ferrets are quick and inquisitive animals, which makes them a joy to own but a challenge to examine. Depending on the way ferrets are raised by their keepers and on individual characteristics, ferrets may be very quiet and relaxed, or inquisitive, stubborn, and even aggressive. In most cases, an ophthalmic examination can be performed by physically restraining the ferret. The common way of restraining ferrets during medical activities is called scruffing and consists of holding the skin on the back of the neck (**Fig. 1**). Depending on the desired positioning, ferrets may be held on a flat surface

Disclosure Statement: The author has nothing to disclose.
[a] Department of Small Animal Medicine and Surgery, UGA Veterinary Medical Center, University of Georgia, 2200 College Station Road, Athens, GA 30602, USA; [b] Tai Wai Small Animal & Exotic Hospital, 75 Chik Shun Street, Tai Wai, Shatin, Hong Kong
* Corresponding author.
E-mail address: kmyrna@uga.edu

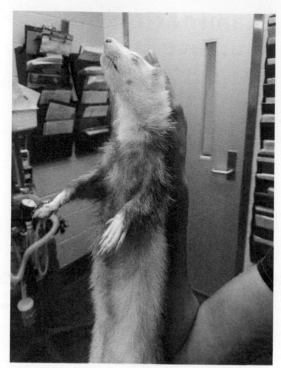

Fig. 1. The scruffing technique for immobilization and examination of the ferret.

or in the air in the so-called hanging position.[1] Holding the back of the neck permits the operators to control the head of the ferret, preventing accidental bites. Also, some ferrets become completely immobile when restrained in this manner.

An alternative to physical restraint is chemical restraint. Chemical restraint is rarely required for a simple ophthalmic examination, including intraocular pressure (IOP) measurement, but may be needed if more invasive diagnostic procedures are performed or if the ferret is especially aggressive.[2] Because specific literature on the effects of most anesthetic drugs on the ocular parameters of ferrets is lacking, effects similar to those demonstrated in other domestic animals should be assumed. For noninvasive ophthalmic testing procedures, the use of midazolam or butorphanol alone is sufficient. The suggested dose for midazolam or butorphanol that provides relaxation sufficient for ophthalmic testing is 0.2 mg/kg intramuscularly for either drug. This is the minimal dose that allows blood pressure measurement from 10 to 20 minutes postinjection in all ferrets, with no side-effects noted except minimal hypothermia.[3]

After the ferret is properly restrained, examination can be accomplished with a combination of direct and oblique illumination of the eye. A direct ophthalmoscope is an excellent tool to examine the corneal surface, as is a transilluminator focused on the eyelid and then used at a 90° angle to illuminate the cornea from the side. This technique backlights the cornea somewhat and helps localize abnormalities to the corneal surface. A normal ferret eye is pictured in **Fig. 2**. Regular ophthalmic diagnostics are also recommended. Schirmer tear tests are cumbersome in the small eye of the ferret but can be accomplished. Normal values have been published as 5.31 mm/min plus or minus 1.32 mm.[4] Fluorescein stain can be used to evaluate for corneal defects by placing a wetted strip to the sclera or a drop of mixed fluorescein solution on the

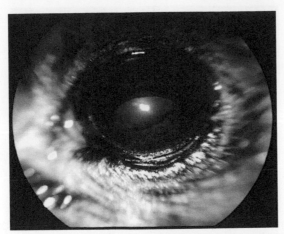

Fig. 2. A normal ferret eye. Note the elliptical pupil and domed cornea. (*Courtesy of* Christa Corbett, DVM, DACVO, Latham, NY.)

cornea. Rinsing may be necessary to determine true stain uptake. IOP readings are published for the applanation tonometer Tono-Pen (Reichert Technologies, Depew, NY) as 14 mm Hg plus or minus 3.27 mm Hg.[4] The TonoVet (Icare, Finland, Oy), a rebound tonometer well-suited to the small size of the ferret eye, has published normal values of 14.07 mm Hg plus or minus 0.35.[2] When applanation and rebound tonometers were compared in the same ferret population, there was poor agreement between these instruments (95% of the results differed between −20.8 and +23.8 mm Hg) and applanation tonometry was less consistent. Multiple factors need to be accounted for in ferrets when measuring IOP because a difference between male and female sex, and a circadian trend (with lower IOP found at night) have been found.[2]

Conjunctivitis

Ferrets housed with improper bedding can develop a conjunctivitis caused by dust and debris.[5] This conjunctivitis is bilateral and accompanied by the presence of debris in the tear film. This can be appreciated by illuminating the eye from the side and looking for irregularity on the corneal surface, followed by fluorescein staining to rule out corneal ulceration. Conjunctivitis has also been reported in association with systemic disease. Most notably, canine distemper presents with ocular signs early in the course of the disease.[6] Canine distemper in the early catarrhal phase is characterized by conjunctivitis, anorexia, fever, and nasal discharge.[7] Ferrets with canine distemper will progress to a pruritic rash followed by hyperkeratosis of the footpads.[8] The disease has poor prognosis and early identification is helpful for patient isolation and client communication (**Fig. 3**).[7]

Human influenza virus infection can mimic canine distemper virus conjunctivitis and should be considered as a rule-out.[7,9,10] Salmonellosis, a notable zoonosis, can present with conjunctivitis, lethargy, vomiting, anorexia, diarrhea, and pale mucous membranes.[11,12] Diagnosis is made by positive fecal culture.[12] *Mycobacterium* infection can result in prominent conjunctival lesions in the disseminated form.[13] A retrospective study of mycobacterial infection in ferrets showed 3 characteristics: eyelid lesions, upper or lower respiratory and gastrointestinal signs, and digestive symptoms.[14] The eyelid lesions in these reports included unilateral or bilateral swelling, edema, or abscess or elevation of the third eyelid, without conjunctival or corneal lesions, which failed to respond to topical antibiotic or steroid treatment.[14] In another report, an affected ferret presented with a proliferative lesion on the third eyelid, whereas another

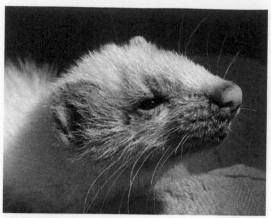

Fig. 3. Ferret distempter conjunctivitis. (*Courtesy of* Nicola Di Girolamo, DMV, MSc (EBHC), PhD, DECZM (Herpetology), Hong Kong.)

presented with conjunctival swelling and serous ocular discharge.[15] Other clinical signs were vague and included cough, weight loss, and depression. Diagnosis is confirmed by detecting the bacteria with cytologic evaluation of conjunctival swabs or histopathologic evaluation of conjunctival biopsies.[13]

Distichiasis, causing epiphora, chronic blepharospasm, and conjunctivitis, has been reported in a ferret.[16] This ferret responded well to surgical treatment of the aberrant cilia with sharp excision of the hair follicle. Chronic ocular discomfort and discharge is an indication for close examination of the eyelid margins for abnormal hairs.

Corneal Disease

The structure of the ferret cornea is similar to other domestic species and is susceptible to corneal surface trauma. Congenital dermoid cysts have been reported in the ferret and have the classic appearance of haired skin on the corneal surface of the eye.[17] Additionally, intraocular disease can result in corneal edema or scar and should be differentiated from corneal surface disease (**Fig. 4**).

The appearance and causes of corneal ulceration in the ferret are similar to other species. Early indications of corneal ulceration include an elevated third eyelid (**Fig. 5**) and corneal edema (**Fig. 6**). After identification of a corneal ulcer, care should

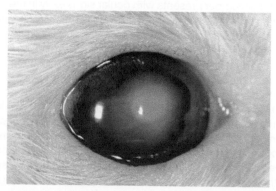

Fig. 4. Focal corneal opacity associated with previous uveitis damaging the corneal endothelium and causing focal scar. Note the irregularity of the iris tissue and dyscoria due to posterior synechia.

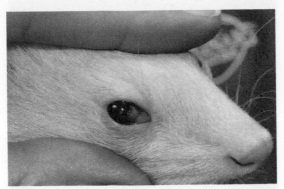

Fig. 5. Elevation of the nictitating membrane in a ferret with ophthalmic disease. (*Courtesy of* Christa Corbett, DVM, DACVO, Latham, NY.)

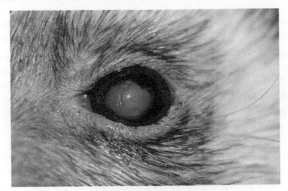

Fig. 6. Diffuse corneal edema and loose epithelium in a ferret with a superficial corneal ulceration. (*Courtesy of* Manuela Crasta, DECVO, Latham, NY.)

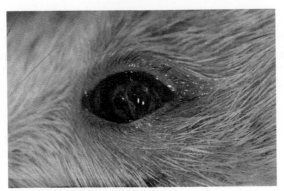

Fig. 7. Perforation of a malacic ulcer in a ferret. Note the protruding fibrin clot and probably iris prolapse temporally. (*Courtesy of* Manuela Crasta, DECVO, Latham, NY.)

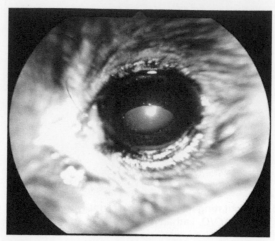

Fig. 8. Corneal pigmentation of unknown cause demonstrated by a spattered appearance of brown spots on the surface of the eye. Corneal pigmentation is typically the result of chronic corneal irritation. (*Courtesy of* Christa Corbett, DVM, DACVO, Latham, NY.)

be taken to ensure the eye is not exophthalmic given that exposure keratitis secondary to an orbital mass effect has been reported.[18] Treatment of superficial corneal ulceration includes topical, broad-spectrum, antimicrobial agents. If the cornea appears infiltrated or has a hazy yellow or malacic appearance, cytologic evaluation and/or culture is indicated. Perforated eyes warrant systemic antimicrobial therapy in addition to topical antimicrobial therapy. A ruptured ulcer has a characteristic protrusion of fibrin or iris or both (**Fig. 7**). Healed ulcers may leave focal corneal scars that present as localized gray or white opacities. Additionally, the ferret cornea can pigment in a patient with pigmentary keratitis of unknown cause (**Fig. 8**).

Lymphoplasmacytic keratitis, an uncommon corneal disease, was reported in a 2-year-old ferret; it was ultimately associated with multicentric lymphoma.[19] The keratitis was unresponsive to topical steroids and the animal did not show systemic signs of disease until 8 weeks after presentation. In a case of systemic coronavirus, the patient presented with lethargy, weight loss, pruritus, and a corneal opacity characterized by a yellow color.[20] The eye demonstrated signs of anterior uveitis in a fashion similar to cats with feline infectious peritonitis.[20]

SUMMARY

Corneal surface disease in the ferret can be a symptom of significant systemic disease and requires a thorough ophthalmic examination to find the underlying cause of any lesions. An examination can be accomplished with a finoff transilluminator and magnification or appropriate use of the direct ophthalmoscope. Many conditions can be successfully managed if properly identified and treated.

REFERENCES

1. Dudás-Györki Z, Szabó Z, Manczur F, et al. Echocardiographic and electrocardiographic examination of clinically healthy, conscious ferrets. J Small Anim Pract 2011;52(1):18–25.
2. Di Girolamo N, Andreani V, Guandalini A, et al. Evaluation of intraocular pressure in conscious ferrets (*Mustela putorius furo*) by means of rebound tonometry and comparison with applanation tonometry. Vet Rec 2013;172(15):396.

3. van Zeeland YRA, Wilde A, Bosman IH, et al. Non-invasive blood pressure measurement in ferrets (*Mustela putorius furo*) using high definition oscillometry. Vet J 2017;228:53–62.
4. Montiani-Ferreira F, Mattos BC, Russ HHA. Reference values for selected ophthalmic diagnostic tests of the ferret (*Mustela putorius furo*). Vet Ophthalmol 2006;9(4):209–13.
5. Moody KD, Bowman TA, Lang CM. Laboratory management of the ferret for biomedical research. Lab Anim Sci 1985;35(3):272–9.
6. Perpinan D, Ramis A, Tomas A, et al. Outbreak of canine distemper in domestic ferrets (*Mustela putorius furo*). Vet Rec 2008;163(8):246–50.
7. Langlois I. Viral diseases of ferrets. Vet Clin North Am Exot Anim Pract 2005;8(1): 139–60.
8. Deem SL, Spelman LH, Yates RA, et al. Canine distemper in terrestrial carnivores: a review. J Zoo Wildl Med 2000;31(4):441–51.
9. Marois P, Boudreault A, DiFranco E, et al. Response of ferrets and monkeys to intranasal infection with human, equine and avian influenza viruses. Can J Comp Med 1971;35(1):71–6.
10. Zitzow LA, Rowe T, Morken T, et al. Pathogenesis of avian influenza A (H5N1) viruses in ferrets. J Virol 2002;76(9):4420–9.
11. Gorham JR, Cordy DR, Quortrup ER. Salmonella infections in mink and ferrets. Am J Vet Res 1949;10(35):183–92.
12. Pignon C, Mayer J. Zoonoses of ferrets, hedgehogs, and sugar gliders. Vet Clin North Am Exot Anim Pract 2011;14(3):533–49.
13. Pollock C. Mycobacterial infection in the ferret. Vet Clin North Am Exot Anim Pract 2012;15(1):121–9, vii.
14. Mentré V, Bulliot C. A retrospective study of 17 cases of mycobacteriosis in domestic ferrets (*Mustela putorius furo*) between 2005 and 2013. J Exotic Pet Med 2015;24(3):340–9.
15. Nakata M, Miwa Y, Tsuboi M, et al. Mycobacteriosis in a domestic ferret (*Mustela putorius furo*). J Vet Med Sci 2014;76(5):705–9.
16. Verboven CAPM, Djajadiningrat-Laanen SC, Kitslaar W-JP, et al. Distichiasis in a ferret (*Mustela putorius furo*). Vet Ophthalmol 2014;17(4):290–3.
17. Ryland LM, Gorham JR. The ferret and its diseases. J Am Vet Med Assoc 1978; 173(9):1154–8.
18. McBride M, Mosunic CB, Barron GHW, et al. Successful treatment of a retrobulbar adenocarcinoma in a ferret (*Mustela putorius furo*). Vet Rec 2009;165(7): 206–8.
19. Ringle MJ, Lindley DM, Krohne SG. Lymphoplasmacytic keratitis in a ferret with lymphoma. J Am Vet Med Assoc 1993;203(5):670–2.
20. Lindemann DM, Eshar D, Schumacher LL, et al. Pyogranulomatous panophthalmitis with systemic coronavirus disease in a domestic ferret (*Mustela putorius furo*). Vet Ophthalmol 2016;19(2):167–71.

Ocular Surface Diseases in Marine Mammals

Carmen Maria Helena Colitz, DVM, PhD, DACVO[a,b,*]

KEYWORDS

- Cornea • Keratopathy • Ulcer • Lens • Cataract • Pinniped • Cetacean

KEY POINTS

- Marine mammals' eyes are adapted for sight and physiologic health in both the water and air environments.
- Marine mammals' adnexa have adaptations for these functions, including lack of the lipid tear film layer and nasolacrimal apparatus.
- The most common corneal diseases in dolphins are medial keratopathy, horizontal keratopathy, and axial keratopathy.
- The most common ophthalmologic diseases in pinnipeds are pinniped keratopathy and cataracts.

INTRODUCTION

The eyes of marine mammals are adapted for both sight and physiological health under water as well as on land. Ophthalmic lesions in marine mammals, both in the wild and in human care, often affect the cornea, and less often the adnexa. Despite affecting similar ocular structures, the underlying causes are different. Marine mammals in the wild are more likely to develop lesions due to trauma,[1–3] whereas, marine mammals in human care are more often affected by environmental factors.[3–6] Regardless of the cause of disease, the ocular surface of any eye has certain requirements to maintain its overall health and transparency to allow functional sight.

The physical structures important to the health of the ocular surface include the adnexa and the cornea. The adnexal structures include the extraocular muscles and orbital contents, the upper and lower eyelids, the third eyelid, the nasolacrimal system, and the conjunctiva. The normal cornea is an immunologically privileged site due to its lack of vascularization and lymphatics.[7] The health of the adnexa and the cornea are

Disclosure Statement: Disclosure of any relationship with a commercial company that has a direct financial interest in subject matter or materials discussed in article or with a company making a competing product, None.
a Ophthalmology Department, All Animal Eye Care, Inc, 505 Commerce Way, Jupiter, FL 33458, USA; b Department of Molecular Biomedical Sciences, North Carolina State University, 1060 William Moore Drive, Raleigh, NC 27607, USA
* 505 Commerce Way, Jupiter, FL 33458.
E-mail address: ccolitzacvo@gmail.com

closely tied. Normal anatomy and function of the eyelids is important as the eyelids keep the precorneal tear film properly spread over the corneal and conjunctival surfaces. Reflex blinking and tearing helps to clear debris and foreign bodies. In addition, numerous factors at the cellular and molecular level contribute to a healthy ocular surface environment. These include a functional and balanced precorneal tear film, as well as the ability to control the innate and adaptive immune responses via tolerance and modulatory mechanisms following oxidative stress and/or microbial insults. Finally, a healthy ocular surface also needs a balance of anti-inflammatory proteins and hormones including interleukin-1 and transforming growth factor-ß.[8] The balance is so delicate that any environmental, microbial, genetic, or other similar factor can activate the ocular surface immune system. Inflammation of any type negates the innate immunologic privilege, and ingrowth of corneal vascularization allows lymphatics to enter the cornea.[8] Further complicating matters is the possibility of corneal nerve damage during nonspecific keratopathy. Either hyperalgesia or hypoalgesia, due to corneal nerve dysfunction, would exacerbate clinical signs. Hyperalgesia would manifest with signs of excessive pain despite minimal obvious signs of keratopathy; and, corneal nerve dysfunction may allow unobserved corneal damage due to lack of obvious signs of pain.[9]

ANATOMIC AND PHYSIOLOGIC DIFFERENCES OF THE ADNEXA AND CORNEA

The overall structure of the cetacean and pinniped globe is similar to those of terrestrial mammals; however, there are some important functional differences.[10] The pinniped globe is large, which decreases the curvature of the cornea. Although the cetacean globe is not as large, the anterior segment is flattened, resulting in a similar decrease in corneal curvature. Both cetacean and pinniped corneas are thinner axially and thicker peripherally.[10,11] Similar to cetaceans, the pinniped corneal layers from external to internal include the epithelium, Bowman layer, a thick collagenous stroma that is thicker peripherally than axially, Descemet membrane, and the endothelium.[10,11] Most cetacean species have a Bowman layer, and, it is much thicker than that of pinnipeds. Most pinniped species have a flattened plateau located just inferonasal to the axial cornea, making them capable of focusing incoming light through the stenopeic pupil directly to the area centralis.[11,12]

Cetaceans and pinnipeds spend a significant amount of their lives in the water, altering the need for some adnexal structures. The nasolacrimal secretory and excretory system differs from terrestrial mammal systems. They do not have a nasolacrimal drainage system. In addition, their precorneal tear film is different from that of terrestrial mammals, which have 3 layers; that is, the lipid layer, the aqueous layer, and the mucin layer. Pinnipeds clinically and histologically lack meibomian glands, and this is consistent with lacking the lipid layer of the precorneal tear film.[13] This is true in cetaceans as well (Colitz and R.R. Dubielzig, unpublished data, 2018). Both cetaceans and pinnipeds, however, have a significantly thicker mucin layer in their tear film compared with terrestrial mammals. Mucins in the preocular tear film are vital to the protection of the ocular surface, as they protect against pathogens and likely other challenges that the marine eye faces in the aquatic environment. Cetacean tears have been found to have a variety of mucins, as well as lysozyme and albumin.[14] The tear film from 2 dolphin species evaluated has been shown to inhibit the growth of the bacteria *Escherichia coli*,[15] strongly suggesting the antimicrobial function of the mucins. In the most detailed study to date, it was found that the carbohydrate-to-protein ratio of pinnipeds was the most similar to that of humans, although each species had a unique profile.[16] Although the precorneal tear film of marine mammals is still under investigation, enough data have been gathered to understand that it is of critical importance for the health of the ocular surface.

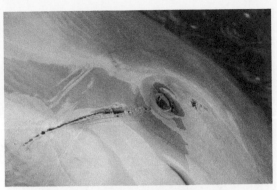

Fig. 1. Right side of face of an Atlantic bottlenose dolphin (*Tursiops truncatus*) with a traumatic skin laceration that begins above the right eye, has a small upper eyelid laceration medially, and continues ventrally to below the level of the mouth.

EYELID LESIONS
Cetaceans

Eyelid lesions in cetaceans are uncommon; however, traumatic eyelid lacerations may occur from rough play or fighting (**Fig. 1**). If severe, they can be surgically repaired. Eyelid hyperemia is relatively common when keratopathy is painful due to self-trauma. Eyelid masses are rare but have been diagnosed (**Fig. 2**). Depigmentation of the eyelid margins occurs in walruses as they age.

Pinnipeds

The eyelids of pinnipeds do not typically develop congenital anomalies; although one animal, thus far, has been identified with a congenital adhesion or lack of separation at the medial aspect of the superior eyelid to the adjacent margin of nictitating membrane. This impeded the normal movement of the third eyelid, and surgical correction was performed, allowing proper movement.[6] Eyelid masses have been identified and diagnosed in many phocid and otariid species (**Fig. 3**). Trauma, usually from playing or fighting with exhibit mates, is not uncommon. Most traumatic eyelid injuries heal

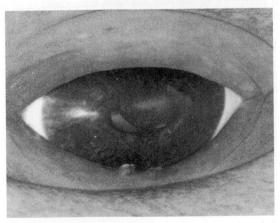

Fig. 2. Left eye (OS) of an Atlantic bottlenose dolphin (*T truncatus*) with 2 small raised eyelid margin masses. The cornea also has a horizontal gray linear opacity, horizontal keratopathy. The white lesions medially are artifacts.

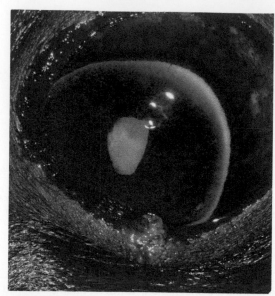

Fig. 3. Left eye (OS) of a South African fur seal (*Arctocephalus pusillus*) with a pink corrugated raised mass on the lower eyelid margin. The eye has numerous lesions, including limbal hyperemia, conjunctival pigment is encroaching on the limbus, perilimbal edema extends into the adjacent cornea, there are 2 oval areas of stromal loss dorsolateral to the axial cornea, and the lens is cataractous.

without surgical intervention.[6] South American sea lions develop chronic dermatitis that can include the periocular skin (**Fig. 4**). The disease is not well understood in terms of etiology, and many possibilities include water temperature, or other environmental factors (Dr Michael Walsh, personal communication, 2016).

CONJUNCTIVAL ISSUES
Cetaceans

Conjunctivitis as a primary disease has not been diagnosed in cetaceans; however, conjunctival hyperemia, chemosis, or excessive proliferation can occur. Hyperemia

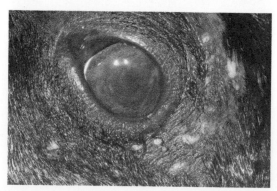

Fig. 4. Left eye (OS) of a South American sea lion (*Otaria flavescens*) with dermatitis as well as stage 1 pinniped keratopathy. The periocular skin has multifocal pale pink skin lesions. The eye has pigment migrating over the medial limbus as well as perilimbal edema.

and chemosis are usually associated with active keratopathy. Severely swollen and proliferative conjunctiva without active keratopathy has been identified, although a specific etiologic cause was not found (**Fig. 5**).

Pinnipeds

Similar to cetaceans, pinnipeds rarely develop primary conjunctivitis. The conjunctiva will become hyperemic with keratopathy or anterior lens luxation. The conjunctiva can become depigmented with chronic keratopathy as well, especially in the walrus.

CORNEAL ISSUES
Cetaceans

Common corneal diseases affecting cetaceans under human care have been recently described in a worldwide epidemiologic study and include medial and temporal keratopathy, horizontal keratopathy, and axial keratopathy.[3] These 4 entities are consistent in their presentation, and more than one of these diseases can occur at the same time.

Medial keratopathy

In a recent worldwide epidemiologic study, the most common corneal disease of cetaceans, medial keratopathy, occurred in 53.9% of animals, and was bilateral in 46.1% of animals.[3] Initially, the pigment medial to the medial limbus begins to migrate toward the adjacent limbus, crossing the limbus and entering the cornea. Once pigment has established itself across the limbus, gray-white corneal fibrosis follows, along with vascularization (see **Fig. 2**). Over time, the lesion can extend to the axial cornea, joining horizontal or axial keratopathy, if present. Uncomplicated medial keratopathy is not painful, often an incidental finding, and may be directly related to excessive UV exposure via the Coroneo effect,[17] similar to pterygium in humans. These lesions are more common in animals with higher UV index (Colitz, personal observation). A large epidemiologic study is under way to evaluate this hypothesis. On rare occasions, a small abscess may develop within the medial keratopathy lesion causing severe pain and cellular infiltrates. Supportive care leads to resolution. Overall, diminished exposure to excessive UV radiation combined with daily UV-protective antioxidant support appears to diminish progression of this disease (Colitz, personal observation).

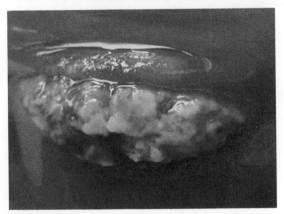

Fig. 5. Left eye (OS) of a Pacific bottlenose dolphin (*Tursiops truncatus gilli*) with severe proliferative conjunctivitis. The conjunctiva of the upper eyelid is severely swollen with thick mucopurulent discharge, possibly a diphtheritic membrane. The eyelid skin has an irregular surface and its margin is not smooth.

Temporal keratopathy

The less common temporal keratopathy is similar to medial keratopathy in presentation but occurs, as its name suggests, at the temporal conjunctiva, limbus, and cornea (**Fig. 6**). Temporal keratopathy occurred in 6.1% of animals and was bilateral in 5.6% of animals.[3] Interestingly, temporal keratopathy appears more common at higher latitudes, whereas medial keratopathy is more common nearer the equator (Colitz and Elisa, personal observation). The Coroneo effect is thought to also cause temporal keratopathy because the eyes of cetaceans are very prominent and UV light can enter from either the medial or lateral aspects as they surface for feeding and other interactions.[17]

Horizontal keratopathy

Horizontal keratopathy is the only entity that can be transient in its initial occurrences. Horizontal keratopathy occurred in 22.8% of animals and 15.6% had bilateral lesions.[3] This disease has been observed in animals younger than 1 year. Typical lesions occur where the superior and inferior eyelids appose. Lesions can be of any length, may be more medial or temporal than perfectly axial, and may be straight, jagged, or irregular (**Fig. 7**A). Either of these lesions can appear and disappear within a 24-hour to 48-hour time period, or be more gradual in improvement. Over time, with repetitive insults, the lesions become permanent; and, there can be new lesions overlying the chronic lesions (**Fig. 7**B). Histologically, the inner corneal epithelial cells invade the Bowman layer, and eventually penetrate this basement membrane structure to invade the anterior corneal stroma.[18]

Predisposing factors of horizontal keratopathy appear to be any nonspecific oxidative stress, including increases in UV exposure or index, use of oral quinolone antibiotics for extended periods of time, and changes in water quality variables. Currently, there is no specific treatment for the initial onset of the disease; however, some of the current approaches include oral UV-protective antioxidants, including grapeseed extract, lutein, and astaxanthin, as well as the use of topical tacrolimus ophthalmic drops. Additionally, providing more shade will help the lesions to lessen more rapidly (Colitz, personal observation).

Axial keratopathy

Axial keratopathy occurred in 24.4% of animals and was bilateral in 11.7% of cases. Clinically, the classic axial keratopathy lesion appears as a pinpoint gray-white opacity

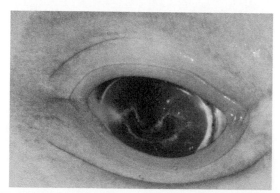

Fig. 6. Right eye (OD) of an Atlantic bottlenose dolphin (*T truncatus*) with temporal keratopathy. There is a triangular gray opacity that originates lateral to the limbus and extends in a triangular shape into the lateral quarter of the cornea. The medial limbus has mild hyperemia and mild pigment migration.

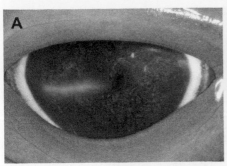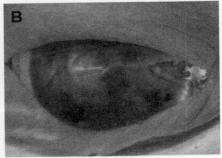

Fig. 7. (*A*) Right eye (OD) of an Atlantic bottlenose dolphin (*T truncatus*) with a horizontal gray linear opacity consistent with horizontal keratopathy. (*B*) Right eye (OD) of an Atlantic bottlenose dolphin (*T truncatus*) with diffuse corneal fibrosis, medial keratopathy, and a thin short axial horizontal gray opacity overlying the more chronic lesions.

in the anterior stroma and typically occurs axially (**Fig. 8**). The opacity may have a less dense gray halo surrounding the dense pinpoint opacity, and it may remain stable for months to a few years. The lesion is not painful in its quiescent state; however, secondary infection with opportunistic organisms causes the lesion to enlarge, often with stromal loss, and results in signs of mild to severe pain when the infection is active.

With chronicity, axial keratopathy and horizontal keratopathy may coexist. Regardless, chronic axial/horizontal keratopathy can encompass most of the axial cornea with a relatively horizontal irregularly rectangular shape. Chronic horizontal keratopathy lesions have a smooth surface, can have variable stromal loss, and often appear to have a rust or brownish hue (**Fig. 9**). When quiescent, there are no signs of obvious pain; however, there can be intermittent episodes of blepharospasm and photophobia. During these flare-ups, lesions may appear the same, have more diffuse edema, or even develop either ulcerative lesions or abscess formation within or at the edges of the lesion.

Predisposing factors of axial keratopathy are not definitively known; however, imbalances in water quality and excessive exposure to UV light are hypothetical etiologies. Unfortunately, this entity does not resolve, and progresses at a variable rate. Secondary infection with opportunistic organisms makes the lesions progress more rapidly. Treatment for active axial keratopathy is described at the end of this article.

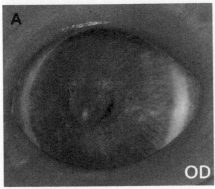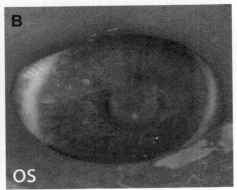

Fig. 8. (*A,B*) Both eyes (OU) of an Atlantic bottlenose dolphin (*T truncatus*) with early axial keratopathy. Each eye has a very small gray pinpoint opacity axially.

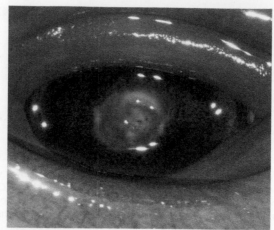

Fig. 9. Left eye (OS) of an Atlantic bottlenose dolphin (*T truncatus*) with chronic axial keratopathy. There is pigment migration over both the medial and lateral limbus and axially there is an irregularly round lesion that is outlined by a rust-colored rim. The center of the lesion has an irregular surface with rust and gray coloration. Surrounding the axial round lesion is a gray outer rim and diffuse blue-gray opacity that is edema.

Traumatic keratopathy

Dolphins are very interactive with their enclosure-mates. This can cause sharp and blunt traumatic events that affect the eyelids and/or corneas. Corneal lacerations may sometimes have concomitant eyelid lacerations that line up with each other. Sometimes, an animal will present with closed eyelids and may or may not have an associated eyelid bruise. An eyelid bruise does not always correlate with corneal damage. Unfortunately, if left untreated in the early stages, a corneal ulcer can become infected with opportunistic organisms (ie, bacteria and/or fungi or yeast) and is at risk for progression and possible corneal perforation. It is the author's opinion that treatment with a combination of either oral ciprofloxacin or enrofloxacin for 5 to 10 days (ie, until the eye begins to open) and doxycycline has diminished the incidence of severe corneal damage, scarring, and perforation. The use of quinolone antibiotics is to combat the aggressive and stromal malacia-causing *Pseudomonas* spp that can quickly lead to corneal perforation. The basis for the use of doxycycline is that it has important inhibitory effects on matrix metalloproteinase-9 (MMP9), as well as immunomodulatory, anti-inflammatory, and prohealing effects.[19–21] MMP9 is the enzyme released by certain bacteria (*Pseudomonas* and *Beta-streptococcus*), by neutrophils, and by keratocytes and is responsible for corneal stromal loss.[22] Once the eyelids begin to open and allow visualization of the lesions, if present, then more a targeted therapeutic plan can be designed and the oral quinolone antibiotics can be discontinued, as they can also cause horizontal keratopathy when used for an extended period.

Pinnipeds

Pinniped keratopathy

Pinniped keratopathy is a well-described and characterized disease affecting all species of pinnipeds, in human care, evaluated to date.[5,6,23] In a recent worldwide epidemiologic study, keratopathy was shown to affect 56.7% of pinnipeds, 51.4% bilaterally affected.[4] The significant risk factors identified included UV index greater than 6, lighter or reflective pool paint colors, being older than 10 years, water salinity less than 29 ppm, having had previous ocular disease, having had previous trauma or injury, and having been tested for Leptospirosis.[4]

The UV index is defined by the US Environmental Protection Agency and is a numerical forecast of the expected risk of overexposure to sunlight.[24] A UV index of 6 to 7 indicates a high risk of sun-related damage without the use of sunblock or a wide-brimmed hat for humans. Facilities that are farther away from the equator have a lower UV index, but those in warmer climates can have UV indices of 10 or 11 for months at a time. UV index does not only mean the actual UV index of the facility's location. The UV index of the pool and enclosure can be affected by the amount of shade the animals have access to and actually use, as well as the color of the dry walls and floors surrounding the pools. Pool colors that are darker or not reflective lower the risk of keratopathy, and also lower the UV index of that pool. Longer days during late spring through early fall can cause cumulative UV damage, even in areas with lower a UV index. Therefore, as animals age, they will continue to accumulate damage related to UV exposure. Feeding the animals and training interactions should try to avoid direct sunlight or try to cover these areas with UV-protective materials.

Salinity was the only water quality parameter identified as a risk factor for keratopathy in the worldwide study. The pH of the water, specifically higher than 7.6, was associated with lower incidence of keratopathy.[4] There may be other water quality variables that are important as well, because corneal edema and blepharospasm occur when parameters become imbalanced. Regardless, it is important to monitor the life support system closely for all changes, even minor ones, as eyes with keratopathy are far more sensitive than normal eyes (Colitz, personal observation). Saltwater pools are ideal, although expensive to maintain. Although not significant in the worldwide study, animals in freshwater were more likely to be affected by keratopathy.[4] This was also shown in a study by Dunn and colleagues in 1996.[25] Other important factors include water temperature, type of disinfection system, creation of by-products of disinfection, environmental pollution, source of the water, and others.[4] One other parameter that is not always evaluated is ammonia. There have been cases of keratopathy where the ammonia had become elevated, then when resolved, affected eyes improved significantly (Colitz, personal observation).

Thus far, pinniped keratopathy has not been identified in pinnipeds in the wild. There are mild variations in clinical presentation of keratopathy between species. One detail is consistent; that is, once keratopathy occurs, the cornea never returns to its original normal state. In addition, a cornea that has or has had keratopathy will be more sensitive to changes in the environmental variables than a normal cornea.

There are 3 stages of clinical keratopathy. Each species has unique differences. Stage 1 affects less than 10% of the cornea and initially presents with mild perilimbal edema, as well as edema just dorsolateral to the axial cornea in some species (**Figs. 10**A, **11**A, and **12**A). Some may have mild pigment migrating across the limbus and/or a small superficial corneal ulcer. Clinical signs of pain are variable and most consistently present with a corneal ulcer. The onset of stage 1 is almost always due to a change in 1 or more environmental factors (Colitz, personal observation). Once identified, the factor or factors should be addressed and corrected, if possible. The corneal ulcer also should be treated with topical antibiotics and pain medications. See section on treatment later in this article.

Stage 2 involves 10% to 20% of the cornea and has either an indolent corneal ulcer or abscess, as well as perilimbal edema, limbal hyperemia, and pigment migration obscuring the limbus (**Figs. 10**B, **11**B, and **12**B). There may or may not be numerous superficial and variably sized corneal bullae. When ulceration is present, there is a consistent indolent component with the epithelium being easy to debride.

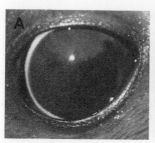
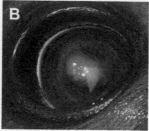
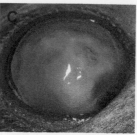

Fig. 10. (A) Stage 1 pinniped keratopathy. Right eye (OD) of a California sea lion (*Zalophus californianus*) with faint perilimbal edema and a gray diffuse superficial corneal opacity located lateral to dorsolateral to the axial cornea. (B) Stage 2 pinniped keratopathy. Right eye (OD) of a California sea lion (*Z californianus*) with perilimbal edema, pigment migration into and attenuating the limbus, and a diffuse gray corneal opacity with an irregular surface. (C) Stage 3 pinniped keratopathy. Right eye (OD) of a California sea lion (*Z californianus*) with completely attenuated limbus, diffuse gray corneal opacity that has patches of denser opacity and an obvious indolent ulcer located dorsomedial to the axial cornea. Most of the corneal surface is irregular.

Unfortunately, this is not practical, as the intense pain does not make the debridement straightforward, and sedation or anesthesia may be risky. Stromal loss occurs with chronicity most likely due to prolonged infection and exposure to UV radiation. In addition, vascularization does not grow as significantly as in other species; thus, making healing a very slow and painstaking process. Opportunistic infection with bacteria and/or fungi or yeast are part of the progression from stage 1 to stage 2, and eventually stage 3 in some cases.

Stage 3 can encompass from approximately 20% to 100% of the cornea (**Figs. 10**C, **11**C, and **12**C). As said, stage 3 is due to the progression of an opportunistic infection and is extremely aggressive. If not controlled aggressively, progression to full-thickness abscess formation, stromal malacia, extensive stromal loss, descemetocele formation, or even corneal perforation may occur (**Fig. 13**). Surgical repair using

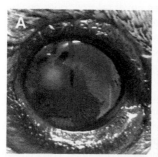
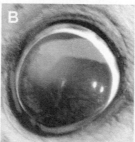
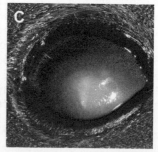

Fig. 11. (A) Stage 1 pinniped keratopathy. Right eye (OS) of a harbor seal (*Phoca vitulina*) that has an oval superficial gray corneal opacity located lateral to the axial cornea. The eye is not held completely open due to blepharospasm. (B) Stage 2 pinniped keratopathy. Right eye (OS) of a harbor seal (*P vitulina*) that has an oval diffuse gray corneal opacity. The limbus is still evident dorsally and medially, but laterally there is pigment migration starting to attenuate the limbus. There is also a cataract. (C) Stage 3 pinniped keratopathy. Right eye (OS) of a harbor seal (*P vitulina*) with diffuse corneal edema with numerous superficial epithelial bullae.

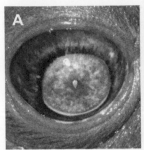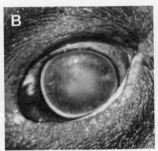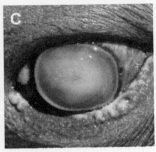

Fig. 12. (A) Stage 1 pinniped keratopathy. Right eye of a walrus (*Odobenus rosmarus*) with pigment migration attenuating most of the limbus. The lower eyelid is beginning to lose pigmentation. (B) Stage 2 pinniped keratopathy. Right eye (OS) of a walrus (*O rosmarus*) that has diffuse gray opacity involving approximately 20% of the axial cornea. There is perilimbal edema and the conjunctival pigment is migrating across the limbus attenuating it dorsally and medially. The lateral conjunctiva has an area where it has lost pigmentation. The lower eyelid is also losing pigmentation. (C) Stage 3 pinniped keratopathy. Right eye (OS) of a walrus (*O rosmarus*) that has diffuse corneal edema encompassing the entire cornea. It is slightly clearer around the peripheral cornea and there are few superficial variably sized epithelial bullae. The lateral conjunctiva has an area of pigment loss. The lower eyelid has an irregular surface and is depigmenting.

BioSIS or amniotic membrane graft with a conjunctival pedicle flap has been used to address deep ulcers or perforations along with lensectomy when cataract or anterior lens luxation is a concurrent problem.[26] Episcleral subconjunctival cyclosporine implants are also placed at the same time or at any anesthetic opportunity to help control keratopathy. See later in this article for details.

All of the stages can attain quiescence, that is, become comfortable, corneal edema improves significantly, ulceration may heal, infection is controlled. Three key details need to be addressed for keratopathy in both pinnipeds and cetaceans to become controlled. First, it is imperative to control the environmental variables that are imbalanced. Second and third are control of the infection and supporting proper

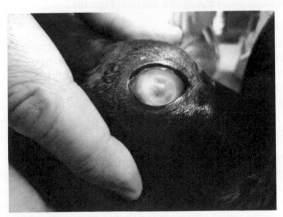

Fig. 13. Stage 3 pinniped keratopathy. Right eye (OD) of a California sea lion (*Z californianus*) with a large malacic corneal ulcer with extensive stromal loss that appears over 85% deep in the central area. There is 3 to 4 mm of corneal vascularization growing in from the limbus extending from 9 o'clock to 1 o'clock.

epithelialization of an ulcer, if present. However, the indolent component often makes control of the disease frustrating in many cases. The use of aggressive epithelial debridement along with burr keratotomy has improved healing of the indolent ulcer component of pinniped keratopathy.

Otariid keratopathy
Keratopathy was initially described in otariids,[23] but, it was soon realized that all species evaluated were similarly affected. The initial description included 100 California sea lions, one Guadalupe fur seal, one northern fur seal, 7 brown fur seals, and 6 Steller sea lions. It was noted that all age groups of otariids could be affected, even as young as 6 months old. The more recent study that included 229 sea lions and fur seals found the incidence to be 51.1%.[4]

In general, the initial lesion in a sea lion occurs dorsolateral to the axial cornea as a focal gray opacity or superficial corneal ulcer. There is also very mild to moderate perilimbal corneal edema, and pigmentation crossing the limbus. The pigment migration makes the limbus appear to attenuate (see **Fig. 10**C).

Phocid keratopathy
Keratopathy in phocids, or true seals, had an incidence of 51.4% in a recent worldwide epidemiologic study.[4] This incidence is similar to that of otariids. Harbor seals are the most numerous of the phocid species in human care. Harp seals are not as numerous as harbor seals, but both species develop corneal lesions similar to California sea lions, that is, perilimbal edema, attenuation of the distinct limbus via pigment migration, and dorsolateral paraxial corneal gray opacities consistent with fibrosis as well as bullae, ulcers, or abscesses (see **Fig. 11**C). Hawaiian monk seal keratopathy includes extensive loss of the epibulbar conjunctival pigment, patchy migration of the pigment that crosses the adjacent limbus, and mild vascularization that crosses the limbus into the adjacent cornea. With chronicity, the corneal opacity becomes dense with severe corneal edema and fibrosis.

Gray seals have the most aggressive keratopathy of all the pinniped species. They develop limbal hyperemia, and vascularization is seen to cross the limbus into the adjacent cornea. The cornea develops dense corneal edema and fibrosis along with chalky white corneal opacity, and the pigmentation that crosses the limbus can progress to involve most or even the entire cornea (**Fig. 14**).

Walrus keratopathy
There are few walrus in human care, but they are the most affected by keratopathy with an incidence of 62.5%. Similar to all species, perilimbal edema, limbal hyperemia, and pigmentation that crosses the limbus are consistent findings (see **Fig. 12**). Their initial corneal lesion is a relatively small axial diffuse gray opacity. Corneal ulcer or abscess formation is common as well. With chronicity, the opacity will encompass a significant portion of the cornea, or even the entire cornea, and conjunctival depigmentation is also common.

Juvenile California sea lion keratopathy
A unique variant of keratopathy affects California sea lions that are approximately 2 to 3 years of age. Juvenile keratopathy causes an acute onset of diffuse corneal edema with few to numerous variably sized bullae (**Fig. 15**). This entity has been identified only in animals on the Pacific coast of the United States or one animal that was transported from California to the east coast. Gradual resolution can take up to 1 year. Supportive care with broad-spectrum topical and oral antibiotics to address opportunistic bacteria and yeast/fungi, as well as oral nonsteroidal anti-inflammatory medications, and

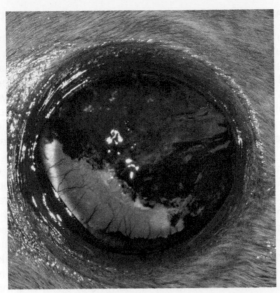

Fig. 14. Left eye (OS) of a gray seal (*Halichoerus grypus*) with severe stage 3 pinniped keratopathy. Most of the cornea is covered with dense pigmentation. The ventrolateral aspect of the cornea has active vascularization and diffuse edema. The limbus has pigment migration over most of the limbal areas.

tramadol for pain. Once controlled and resolving or resolved, it is suggested to use topical 2% cyclosporine or 0.02% or 0.03% tacrolimus twice daily.[6] This has subjectively delayed the onset of pinniped keratopathy as the animal ages (Colitz, personal observation).

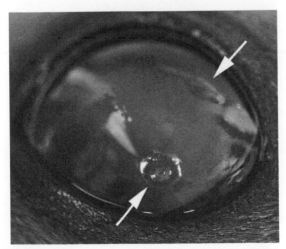

Fig. 15. Left eye (OS) of a California sea lion (*Z californianus*) with juvenile keratopathy. There is diffuse corneal edema with 1 moderately large sized bullae etc (*upper arrow*) and ventrolaterally, there is an irregularly round corneal ulcer with approximately 25% stromal loss (*lower arrow*). There are a few tiny bullae evident dorsomedial to the lower ulcer.

TREATMENT OF ACTIVE KERATOPATHY IN CETACEANS AND PINNIPEDS

The goal of treating pinniped keratopathy is to identify and correct the environmental factor(s) that initiated the flare up, to treat the disease with antibiotics that address the common opportunistic bacteria (*Pseudomonas* spp and coliforms), and provide anti-inflammatory and pain medications. The author's recommendation for initial treatment regimen includes the use of topical 0.1% doxycycline or oral doxycycline to aid in healing and provide some anti-inflammatory effects, as well as topical tobramycin and neomycin-polymyxin-gramicidin ophthalmic drops used 3 times to 4 times a day. The combination of tobramycin, which addresses *Pseudomonas* spp, and neo-polygram, which addresses many coliforms, is a good first-choice combination for the common flora in the aquatic environment. If a fungal or yeast infection is suspected, then either topical 1% voriconazole or 0.1% terbinafine ophthalmic drops used 3 times a day have been practical and less expensive than oral fluconazole or voriconazole, although oral antifungals can be used based on previously published doses.[6] Ideally, collection of cytology and culture samples is suggested but not always practical; therefore, response to therapy may be the only way to monitor progress. Pain control is important. For pinnipeds, either carprofen or meloxicam as the oral nonsteroidal anti-inflammatory medication, and tramadol, if the pain is causing significant blepharospasm and photophobia, are commonly used. Oral meloxicam and/or tramadol are now being use more commonly in cetaceans, although they can be very sensitive to these medications.

TREATMENT OF QUIESCENT KERATOPATHY IN CETACEANS AND PINNIPEDS

Once active lesions have become relatively quiescent, it is important to monitor vigilantly for recurrence. Clinical signs identified and treated quickly are more easily managed; addressing the environmental factor(s) to blame is imperative. The use of topical 2% cyclosporine or 0.02% or 0.03% tacrolimus ophthalmic drops are used

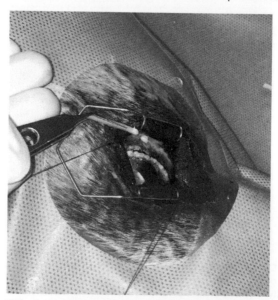

Fig. 16. Right eye (OS) of a harbor seal (*P vitulina*) that underwent lensectomy for cataract and has a small incision where the cyclosporine implant will be placed.

to help control the flare-ups, and episcleral subconjunctival cyclosporine implants have been surgically inserted to help control the disease long-term (**Fig. 16**).[27–29] The implants have provided control for up to 3 or 4 years in some cases where they were placed before onset of keratopathy. Animals with chronic keratopathy may need 2 implants per eye, and the implants may not be helpful for more than 2 years. As mentioned, environmental triggers also need to be eliminated, as much as possible, for ideal control of the disease. Aggressive debridement of the loose corneal epithelium followed by diamond burr keratotomy has improved healing time of the frustrating indolent ulcer component. The corneal ulcers will not heal without debridement of the unadhered epithelial cells. Ulcers that have lost more than one-half to two-thirds of the stroma have benefited from the surgical placement of a conjunctival graft. Deep stromal ulcers, descemetoceles, or perforated corneal ulcers have been addressed using BioSIS graft with conjunctival pedicle flap surgery.[26] Amniotic membrane graft material would be useful beneath the conjunctival pedicle flap as well.

USE OF ANTIOXIDANT SUPPLEMENTS

The author suggests using a variety of antioxidants that include those that are UV-protective as well as those with anti-inflammatory effects. These include grapeseed extract, lutein, lycopene, omega-3-fatty acids, green tea extract (EGCG), vitamin C, vitamin E, milk thistle, and others.[30–35] The chronic exposure to UV, disinfectants, and by-products of disinfection are continually creating free radicals on the skin and corneal surface, including the precorneal tear film. The eye and skin are the most UV-exposed body parts, and in animals that live outside without significant shade, there is obvious damage by a few years of age. Cell damage due to chronic free radical exposure causes keratocyte apoptosis. The cornea absorbs most of the UV entering the eye, making it continually susceptible to free radicals. The normal cornea is rich in endogenous antioxidants, including glutathione peroxidase, glutathione reductase, catalase, and superoxide dismutase.[36] However, repeated exposure to UV light diminishes the endogenous antioxidants, increasing corneal damage as well as keratocyte loss and stromal degeneration.[37] Besides addressing and improving the exposure to exogenous factors in the water and environment, the consistent use of antioxidants may help to diminish oxidative stress in the cornea as well as the skin and body. Numerous studies have shown the benefits of the aforementioned antioxidants, as well as many others, in protecting the cells of the body and reducing the long-term effects of free radical damage.

SUMMARY

In summary, there are a variety of ophthalmic lesions that affect the surface of marine mammals in human care. Environmental issues, especially exposure to excessive UV, are very important for the development and progression of these diseases. The keratopathies of cetaceans and pinnipeds will not improve and become quiescent without identifying and trying to balance all of the potential environmental issues. Rapid diagnosis and appropriate aggressive treatment is of utmost importance in minimizing damage to the ocular surface.

REFERENCES

1. Gerber JA, Roletto J, Morgan LE, et al. Findings in pinnipeds stranded along the central and northern California coast, 1984-1990. J Wildlife Dis 1993;29:423–33.

2. Greig DJ, Gulland FMD, Kreuder C. A decade of live California sea lion (Zalophus californianus) strandings along the central California coast: causes and trends, 1991-2000. Aquatic Mammals 2005;31:11–22.

3. Colitz CMH, Walsh MT, McCulloch SD. Characterization of anterior segment ophthalmologic lesions identified in free-ranging dolphins and those under human care. Journal of Zoo and Wildlife Medicine 2016;47:56–75.

4. Colitz CMH, Saville WJA, Walsh MT, et al. Epidemiologic study of risk factors associated with corneal disease in pinnipeds. J Am Vet Med Assoc, in press.

5. Kern TJ, Colitz CMH. Exotic animal ophthalmology. In: Gelatt KN, Gilger BC, Kern TJ, editors. Veterinary Ophthalmology. 5th edition. Ames (IA): John Wiley & Sons, Inc; 2013. p. 1750–819.

6. Colitz CMH, Bailey JE, Mejia-Fava JC. Cetacean and Pinniped Ophthalmology. In: Dierauf L, Gulland FMD, editors. CRC handbook of marine mammal medicine. 3rd edition. CRC Press Taylor & Francis Group; 2018. p. 517–36.

7. Chauhan SK, Dohlman TH, Dana R. Corneal lymphatics: role in ocular inflammation as inducer and responder of adaptive immunity. J Clin Cell Immunol 2014;5: 1–14.

8. Stern ME, Shaumburg CS, Dana R, et al. Autoimmunity at the ocular surface: pathogenesis and regulation. Mucos Immun 2010;3:425–42.

9. Dawson DG, Ubels JL, Edelhauser HF. Cornea and Sclera. In: Kaufman PL, Alm A, editors. Adler's physiology of the eye. 11th edition. Edinburgh (United Kingdom): Saunders Elsevier; 2011. p. 71–130.

10. Miller S, Samuelson D, Dubielzig R. Anatomic features of the Cetacean Globe. Vet Ophthalmol 2013;16:52–63.

11. Miller SN, Colitz CMH, Dubielzig RR. Anatomy of the California sea lion globe. Vet Ophthalmol 2010;13:63–71.

12. Hanke FD, Dehnhardt G, Schaeffel F, et al. Corneal topography, refractive state, and accomodation in harbor seals (Phoca vitulina). Vision Research 2006;46:837–47.

13. Kelleher Davis R, Doane MG, Knop E, et al. Anatomy of ocular gland morphology and tear composition of pinniped. Vet Ophthalmol 2013;16:269–75.

14. Colitz CMH, Sessler RJ, Green-Church K, et al. Tear film analysis of Orcinus orca. Veterinary Ophthalmology 2007;10:411.

15. Kelleher Davis R, Argueso P. Antimicrobial activity detected in ocular and salivary secretions from marine mammals. Kelleher: Association for Research in Vision Ophthalmology; 2015.

16. Kelleher Davis R, Colitz CMH, Staggs L, et al. Carbohydrate profiles in ocular secretions from cetaceans and pinnipeds. Sausalito (CA): International Association of Aquatic Animal Medicine; 2013.

17. Coroneo MT, Muller-Stolzenburg NW, Ho A. Peripheral light focusing by the anterior eye and the ophthalmohelioses. Ophthalmic Surgery 1991;22:705–11.

18. Colitz CMH, Dubielzig RR, Kelleher Davis R. Horizontal Keratopathy in Dolphins Analogous to Keratoconus in Humans. Annual Conference of the Association for Reserach in Vision and Ophthalmology. Fort Lauderdale, 2012. [E-Abstract: 1111].

19. Van Vlem B, Vanholder R, De Paepe P, et al. Immunomodulating effects of antibiotics: literature review. Infection 1996;24:275–91.

20. Ralph RA. Tetracyclines and the treatment of corneal stromal ulceration: a review. Cornea 2000;19:274–7.

21. Chandler HL, Gemensky-Metzler AJ, Bras ID, et al. In vivo effects of adjunctive tetracycline treatment on refractory corneal ulcers in dogs. J Am Vet Med Assoc 2010;237:378–86.

22. Fukuda K, Ishida W, Fukushima A, et al. Corneal Fibroblasts as Sentinel Cells and Local Immune Modulators in Infectious Keratitis. Int J Molec Sciences 2017;18: E1831.
23. Colitz CMH, Renner MS, Manire CA, et al. Characterization of progressive keratitis in Otariids. Vet Ophthalmol 2010;13:47–53.
24. Agency USEP. UV Index 2016.
25. Dunn JL, Overstrom NA, St Aubin DJ. An epidemiologic survey to determine factors associated with corneal and lenticular lesions in Captive Harbor Seals and California Sea Lions. Annual Meeting of the IAAAM; 1996. p. 108–9.
26. Colitz CMH, Bowman M, Cole G, et al. Surgical repair of a corneal perforation or descemetocele with concurrent lensectomy in three pinnipeds. International Association of Aquatic Animal Medicine 2014.
27. Staggs LA, Colitz CMH, Holmes-Douglas S. The use of subconjunctival cyclosporine implants in a California sea lion (Zalophus californianus) prior to cataract surgery. International Association for Aquatic Animal Medicine 2013.
28. Barachetti L, Rampazzo A, Mortellaro CM, et al. Use of episcleral cyclosporine implants in dogs with keratoconjunctivitis sicca: pilot study. Veterinary Ophthalmology 2015;18:234–41.
29. Colitz CMH, Gilger BC, Grundon R, et al. The use of episcleral subconjunctival cyclosporine implants to control otariid keratopathy. Annual Conference of the International Association of Aquatic Animal Medicine 2016.
30. Chandler HL, Colitz CMH. Protection of canine lens epithelial cells from ultraviolet radiation induced apoptosis with grape seed extract. 41st Annual Meeting of the American College of Veterinary Ophthalmologists; 2010. p. 422.
31. Souyoul SA, Saussy KP, Lupo MP. Nutraceuticals: a review. Dermatol Ther (Heidelb) 2018;8:5–16.
32. Grether-Beck S, Marini A, Jaenicke T, et al. Molecular evidence that oral supplementation with lycopene or lutein protects human skin against ultraviolet radiation: results from a double-blinded, placebo-controlled, crossover study. Br J Dermatol 2016;176:1231–40.
33. Roberts RL, Green J, Lewis B. Lutein and zeaxanthin in eye and skin health. Clin Dermatol 2009;27:195–201.
34. Qin YJ, Chu KO, Yip YW, et al. Green tea extract treatment alleviates ocular inflammation in a rat model of endotoxin-induced uveitis. PLoS One 2014;9: e103995.
35. Svobodova A, Zdarilova A, Maliskova J, et al. Attenuation of UVA-induced damage to human keratinocytes by silymarin. J Dermatol Sci 2007;46:21–30.
36. Buddi R, Lin B, Atilano SR, et al. Evidence of oxidative stress in human corneal disease. J Histochem Cytochem 2002;50:341–51.
37. Newkirk KM, Chandler HC, Parent AE, et al. Ultraviolet radiation-induced corneal degeneration in 129 mice. Toxicol Pathol 2007;35:819–26.

Ocular Surface Disease in Birds

Angela Griggs, DVM, DACVO

KEYWORDS

- Avian • Blepharitis • Conjunctivitis • Keratitis • Ophthalmology

KEY POINTS

- The anatomy and physiology of the avian eye are similar to companion animals; however, some differences require modification of examination expectations and diagnostic technique.
- Diseases of the avian eyelid, conjunctiva, and cornea occur because of a variety of infectious etiologies, many of which may be a manifestation of concurrent systemic disease.
- Noninfectious ocular disease in birds is usually secondary to trauma or poor husbandry. Hereditary ocular disease is infrequent.

INTRODUCTION

Avian ophthalmic anatomy is similar to that of most other species, and similar infectious and noninfectious ocular disease processes have been reported. Surface disease is the focus of this article; therefore, discussion of examination, diagnostics, and treatment will be limited to the eyelid, conjunctiva, tear film, and cornea.

ANATOMY

Similar to companion animals, birds have an upper and lower eyelid, each with a lacrimal punctum draining to a nasolacrimal duct. Although clinical significance is minimal, it is interesting to note that in birds the lower eyelid is more mobile than the upper eyelid. Meibomian glands are absent; however, an inferotemporal orbital lacrimal gland and Harderian gland near the base of the nictitans are present in most reported species.

A nictitating membrane is also present. The nictitating membrane lacks a gland and has voluntary mobility via contracture of the pyramidalis muscle via cranial nerve VI.[1] It advances from dorsomedial to ventrolateral in many species. The membrane can be more transparent in birds compared with companion animals as evident in **Fig. 1**. The

The author has nothing to disclose.
North Houston Veterinary Ophthalmology, 1646 Spring Cypress Road, Suite 116, Spring, TX 77388, USA
E-mail address: AGriggs09@yahoo.com

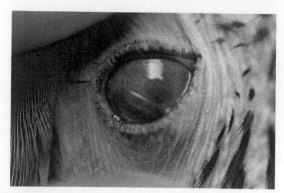

Fig. 1. Example of nictitating membrane transparency.

transparency may be so impressive that the web of vasculature could be mistaken for keratitis if the membrane is persistently elevated by the patient during examination or if it is permanently extruded secondary to symblepharon.[2]

The avian cornea has the same mammalian layers, plus a Bowman-like layer.[3] In addition to deformation of the lens, avian accommodation occurs with changes in corneal curvature. Half or more of the accommodative ability of the chicken and pigeon come from corneal shape changes.[4] The peripheral cornea may be flattened via contraction of Crampton muscle, and is responsible for focusing light on the temporal fovea.[5,6] The refractive power of bald eagle corneas is as high as 40.5 diopters.[7] By comparison, the total (lenticular and corneal) accommodative range of the chicken and pigeon eye is 15- to 17-D.[4]

Regarding evolutionary changes to provide corneal protection from the sun, it was proposed that smaller-eyed birds (eg, pigeon) have less extravagant adnexa (brows and periocular feathering), because the smaller cornea prevents the sun glare from causing significant visual disturbances that may affect foraging or safety. They proposed the converse is true for larger-eyed birds (eg, ostrich), which need exaggerated adnexa to shade the cornea from the sun's glare.[8]

EXAMINATION

Avian ophthalmic examination is similar to other species with few exceptions that will be discussed where applicable. Wild-caught and pet birds that are not well socialized will exhibit variable levels of stress during examination. For this reason, examination should begin with observation of the patient in its natural enclosure when possible. In addition to observation of posture, mentation, and natural movements, there should be a thorough discussion regarding diet, behavior, environment, exposure to other birds, and any pertinent history pertaining to the presenting complaint.

Once the patient is restrained, observe for movement and symmetry of the globes and periocular region. Range of ocular movement varies by species partially dependent on globe shape.[9] If ocular or nasal discharge is present, collection of samples for cytology and culture may be indicated. Standard swab techniques are used for cytology and culture. If signs of upper respiratory disease are present, direct sampling from the nares and choanal slit, and indirect sinus collection via nasal flushing, should be performed. Conjunctival biopsy can also be considered if conjunctivitis is refractory to treatment.

Measurement of tear production can be performed via phenol red thread test, standard Schirmer tear test strip, modified Schirmer tear test strips, or ondodontic paper point test.[10–13] The ability to perform tonometry is limited by the size of the eye. Because of the small surface area of the instrument, utilization of the TonoVet is recommended in avian species with smaller eyes. Lastly, fluorescein staining should be performed in the presence of corneal opacities or if signs of ocular pain are present (blepharospasm, excessive grooming, or guarding of the eye). To aid with precise administration, the fluorescein strip can be placed in a syringe with sterile eye wash and the needle removed from the hub. Fluorescein testing is recommended after completion of the intraocular examination, because a large stained ulcer may obstruct the examiner's view of intraocular structures.

There may be need to modify what is considered a positive menace response when assessing for vision. The traditionally observed blink response to hand motion is inconsistent in birds; therefore, vision is best assessed by observing foraging, object tracking, or avoidance behavior. Some species, such as hummingbirds, may consistently lack a menace response.[14]

Pupillary light reflex (PLR) expectations also vary from companion animal species. When assessing direct PLR, there is often pupillary constriction immediately followed by pupil dilation. This effect can be attributed to voluntary control of the striated iris muscles, and caused by excitement or nervousness in a clinical setting. A consensual PLR should not be expected because of complete decussation of optic nerve fibers at the optic chiasm and after the pretectal nucleus. Despite this anatomic variation in avian species, a consensual PLR can sometimes be observed and is attributed to light penetrating the thin intraorbital septum that separates the globes, leading to stimulation of the contralateral retina.[15]

INFECTIOUS ETIOLOGIES

Numerous bacteria, viruses, fungi, and parasites have been isolated from ocular surface disease. However, it may be difficult to elucidate if the organism is the primary cause for disease. Reported avian ocular pathogens are listed in **Box 1**.

Bacterial

Surveys of conjunctival bacteria in a variety of bird species determined gram-positive bacteria are the most common normal flora among terrestrial birds.[16–19] In most reports, coagulase-negative *Staphylococcus* predominated. The second most common isolate was *Streptococcus* in psittacines and *Corynebacterium* in raptors. A survey of bustards determined *Micrococcus* predominated followed by *Staphylococcus* subspecies.[20] Almost half of the birds, 41% of psittacines and 45% of bustards, had negative bacterial cultures. In tawny owls, coagulase-positive *Staphylococcus* predominated, followed by *Escherichia coli*.[21]

Healthy captive blue-and-gold macaws from Brazil had conjunctival cultures that also revealed gram-positive organisms were most prevalent (49%), but *Bacillus* subspecies were most common, followed by *Staphylococcus* subspecies. There was also a higher fungal detection rate (28%) than previously reported.[12]

The conjunctiva from a single eye from 10 Screech owls was sampled. *Staphylococcus* (coagulase-negative) was cultured from 10 owls. Nine of 46 eyes had nonulcerated corneal opacities.[22]

Coagulase-negative *Staphylococcus* and 1 case of *Staphylococcus aureus* were the only isolates in various raptor species from a zoologic garden. Over 50% of isolates were resistant to most antibiotics tested. Susceptible antibiotics included cefadroxil, cefalexin, cefavecin, oxytetracycline, streptomycin, kanamycin, amikacin, and enrofloxacin.[23]

Box 1
Infectious etiologies of the ocular surface in birds

Bacterial

Staphylococcus

Streptococcus

Clostridium

Erysipelothrix

Mycoplasma

Moraxella

Chlamydophila psittaci

Salmonella

Bordatella

Escherichia coli

Pseudomonas

Actnobacillus

Pasteurella

Mycobacterium

Fungal

Aspergillus

Cladosporium

Rhinosporidium

Scedosporium

Candida

Viral

Avianpox

Herpesvirus

Newcastle disease virus

Paramyxovirus-2

Papovavirus

Papilloma-like virus

Cytomegalovirus

Avian influenza virus

West Nile virus

Reticuloendotheliosis virus

Parasitic

Philophthalmus gralli

Oxyspirura

Ceratospira

Thelazia

Plasmodium

Cryptosporidium

Encephalitozoon hellem

Acanthamoeba

Infrequent surveys of aquatic birds suggest gram-negative bacteria may predominate in these species. In a survey from conjunctiva of healthy ducklings 57% of isolates were Gram stain negative.[24] The most common isolate in conjunctiva of healthy penguins was Corynebacterium, followed by Staphylococcus.[25] In contrast to these reports, Enterococcus subspecies (53%) and other gram-positive cocci (14%) were reported from the conjunctiva in healthy flamingos.[26]

Conjunctivitis is a common presentation of avian ocular disease and maybe a primary or secondary condition. Several infectious and noninfectious causes have been documented.

Infectious etiologies can be associated with respiratory disease or other systemic illness. Clinical findings include conjunctival hyperemia, ocular discharge, and chemosis. Additionally, keratitis or blepharitis may be present.

Fibrinopurulent blepharoconjunctivitis of poultry starting as focal necrosis at the mucocutaneous junction and progressing to complete eyelid necrosis was potentially caused by a combination of Staphylococcus hyicus, E coli, and Streptococcus.[27] A proposed unidentified Staphylococcus cytotoxin may have been necessary for the clinical signs, as neither S hyicus nor E coli caused disease when scarified into eyelid margins. Blepharoconjunctivitis and uveitis caused by Pasteurella multocida were reported.[28]

Extensive investigation of Mycoplasma subspecies in a variety of avian species has been reported since a conjunctivitis outbreak in finches on the East coast in the early 1990s,[29] with new geographic distribution studied as recently as 2018.[30] Mycoplasma has contributed to conjunctivitis with or without keratitis in numerous other species including chickens, blue jays, mockingbirds, starlings, and canaries.[31-35] Successful treatment with topical ciprofloxacin and oral tylosin in water was reported in finches.[36]

Conjunctivitis and hyperkeratotic eyelids leading to blindness secondary to Actinobacillus suis in a Canada goose was reported.[37] Three of 5 waterfowl with systemic Actinobacillus subspecies had matting of periocular feathers, but it was uncertain if the organism was related to the clinical signs.[38]

Numerous ophthalmic cases involving Amazon parrots have been reported. A retrospective study of 57 Amazon parrots reported pathology of the following tissues in descending order: cornea, lens, conjunctiva, eyelid, lacrimal system, retina, sclera, and orbit.[39]

There has been a large report of tetracycline- and chloramphenicol-resistant Staphylococcus causing blepharokeratoconjunctivitis in a flock of Amazon parrots imported into Japan.[40]

Mycobacterium conjunctivitis was reported in 2 emus.[41] Streptococcus and Pasteurella were isolated from keratitis of a Maximilian's parrot that had Mycobacterium in the small intestine.[42]

Bacterial conjunctivitis secondary to Streptococcus subspecies, Erysipelothrix, Clostridium, Mycobacterium, E coli, Pseudomonas, and Bordetella in passerines has been reported.[43] Symblepharon secondary to Salmonella and E coli septicemia was reported in 2 snowy owl chicks.[2] Ulcerative keratitis and corneal perforations in Siberian and whooping crane chicks secondary to *Pseudomonas aeruginosa* were reported.[44]

Chlamydophila psittaci may cause conjunctivitis with or without corneal involvement, and may be local or systemic.[45] *Chlamydophila* associated with conjunctivitis has been reported in ducks.[46]

A case of granulomatous conjunctivitis causing a mass similar histopathologically to a chalazion was reported in a young ostrich. It was uncertain if *Moraxella* subspecies played a role in the inflammatory process.[47] This case report is an example of the necessity of surgical intervention for avian inflammatory masses. Due to the caseous nature of heterophilic infiltrate, medical therapy alone may not be curative.

Viral

Avian pox has been reported in a variety of wild and domestic species.[48–54] It causes conjunctivitis and ocular discharge as one of the earliest clinical signs,[49,55] but can present as facial or periocular proliferative lesions.[51–53] Ulcerative blepharitis and ocular crusts are the most notable signs[49,55]; however, generalized lesions of the body or respiratory tract disease may be present.[56]

Herpesvirus has been identified in numerous avian species. Marek disease typically manifests in uveal tissue first, but has been associated with keratitis later in the disease process in experimentally infected chicks.[57] A novel alphaherpesvirus, Stigid Herpesvirus 1, was reported in the conjunctiva of 2 great horned owls with papillomatous conjunctivitis and chronic superficial ulcerative keratitis treated with a burr keratotomy and topical antiviral medication.[58]

Newcastle disease virus and paramyxovirus 2 causing conjunctivitis in passerine birds was reported.[43] Eyelid petechiae was a rare finding in chicks experimentally infected with Newcastle disease virus.[59] Blepharitis caused by papovavirus from budgerigar eyelids was reported.[60] A papilloma-like virus causing proliferative blepharoconjunctivitis in an African gray parrot was reported.[61] Cytomegalovirus-like infection was suspected to be the cause of conjunctivitis and respiratory disease in Gouldian finches.[62]

Avian influenza virus H5N1 was diagnosed via conjunctival swab of a wild whooper swan in Japan.[63] Although the no human infections have occurred in the United States, it is important to consider the zoonotic potential of avian diseases when handling a systemically ill patient or birds that may have been imported.

West Nile Virus in hawks has been reported to cause chorioretinitis, but no superficial ocular disease has been described.[64] Reticuloendotheliosis virus has been linked to ocular lymphoma in some birds.[65,66]

Fungal

From the conjunctiva of 97 healthy raptor eyes, 2 eyes had positive *Aspergillus* cultures, and 1 eye was positive for *Cladosporium*.[17] Mycotic infections should be considered a differential diagnosis in ocular surface disease. Cases of ocular pathology caused by fungal disease include nodular blepharoconjunctivitis in mute and black swans caused by *Rhinosporidium*,[67] *Scedosporium apiospermum* causing keratitis and uveitis in layer pullets,[68] *Aspergillus*-induced blepharitis and dermatitis in a falcon,[69] *Aspergillus* causing ulcerative keratitis in a blue-fronted Amazon parrot that led to enucleation,[70] and *Aspergillus* causing a yellow corneal plaque in a Khaki Campbell duck.[71] Ophthalmic *Aspergillus* infections have been treated with oral itraconazole, topical miconazole,[69] and oral and topical voriconazole.[71]

Ocular candidiasis has been reported in ducks, budgerigar, a cormorant, a gull, and chickens, causing nodules of the nictitating membrane and conjunctiva, keratitis, and uveitis.[72–75] Successful treatment with oral ketoconazole and topical miconazole was reported.[72]

Parasitic

Ocular parasites in wild and domestic birds maybe incidental findings or cause pathology. **Fig. 2** demonstrates conjunctivitis secondary to parasitism. The most reported parasites are spirurids, nematodes, and trematodes. *Philophthalmus gralli* flukes were identified in ostriches, greater rheas, waterfowl, and other species.[76–78] *Oxyspirura* were recovered from beneath the nictitating membrane of a fulvous owl with no ocular pathology.[79] Histopathologic examination of ocular and periocular tissues of northern bobwhites infected with *Oxyspirura* demonstrated conjunctivitis, keratitis, corneal fibrosis, and inflammatory damage to the lacrimal ducts, lacrimal glands, and Harderian gland.[80,81] This trematode was found in 78% of lesser prairie chickens.[82] *Ceratospira* reportedly caused conjunctivitis and blepharitis in a Wompoo fruit dove that was causing self-trauma to the eye and face for 3 months.[83] Fewer cases of nematodes are reported and include *Thelazia* in a Senegal parrot and a oriental white stork.[84,85] *Plasmodium* has reportedly caused swollen eyelids in canaries and poultry, and drooping eyelids in parakeets.[75,86]

There are a few reports of *Cryptosporidium* causing conjunctivitis in pheasants,[87] a duck,[88] and a peacock,[89] and keratoconjunctivitis in a parakeet,[60] conjunctivitis, corneal edema and bullae, and uveitis in otus owls treated with azithromycin 40 mg/kg orally once daily.[90] A case of *Encephalitozoon hellem* was identified in an umbrella cockatoo based on conjunctival histology after persistent keratoconjunctivitis.[91] Corneal protozoal infection, although uncommon, should be considered a differential for corneal changes. In Turkey, *Acanthamoeba* was identified in almost 17% of deceased wild birds via polymerage chain reaction (PCR). Keratitis was present in 2 cases.[92]

NONINFECTIOUS ETIOLOGIES
Congenital

Reports of congenital diseases of the ocular surface tissues are infrequent. Diagnosis and surgical correction of partial eyelid agenesis in a peregrine falcon were reported.[93]

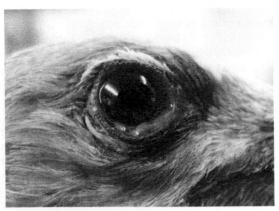

Fig. 2. Parasite-induced conjunctivitis in a laughing gull.

Ectropion has been diagnosed in cockatiels.[94] Congenital symblepharon of unknown cause was reported in a red-vented cockatoo.[72] Suspicion of impatent nasolacrimal ducts was reported in a cockatoo.[94] Bilateral corneal dermoids have been reported in a gosling and a young blue-fronted Amazon.[95,96] The latter were successfully removed via keratectomies.

Traumatic

Surveys of wild and captive birds have demonstrated varying degrees of keratitis, corneal fibrosis, eyelid abnormalities, or other evidence of ocular trauma.[97–101] A survey of wild and captive murres demonstrated 13% of birds had blepharitis or eyelid lacerations; one-third of wild birds had conjunctivitis, and half of the wild birds and 25% of captive birds had corneal fibrosis. Twenty-five percent of wild birds had ulcerative keratitis.[98] In a survey of little owls and scops owls, ocular or periocular trauma-associated lesions were 27.8% and 27.3%, respectively.[99] Another study reported 90% of wild raptors had ocular lesions that could be attributed to trauma.[100] Blunt trauma in birds is more common than penetrating trauma, especially in raptors, and causes significant intraocular damage outside the scope of this article.[101]

Causes and treatment regarding superficial trauma of the eyelids and cornea of birds do not differ significantly from other species (eg, corneal ulcers, conjunctival foreign bodies, or eyelid lacerations). Cytology and culture should be considered, especially if ocular discharge is present. Eyelid abrasions and superficial corneal ulcers should be treated with topical antibiotics until healed. Corneal grafting surgeries can be performed for stromal or malacic ulcers. Penetrating keratoplasty followed by primary corneal closure in 2 great horned owls and followed by placement of donor cornea in 1 great horned owl and 1 California brown pelican was successful in treating bullous keratopathy and dense corneal neovascularization.[102–104]

Nutritional

Eyelid swelling, keratitis, and conjunctivitis are common clinical signs caused by vitamin A deficiency in birds. It is common in birds exclusively fed seeds, especially sunflower seeds. It can also occur because of intestinal, pancreatic, or hepatic disease.[53] Oral or parenteral supplementation is recommended. Vitamin B5 (pantothenic acid) deficiency was reported in Japanese quail and caused conjunctivitis, facial dermatitis, and decreased hatchability.[105]

Neoplastic

Uncommonly, neoplasia of the eyelids, conjunctiva, or orbit, with or without exophthalmia, has been reported.[106–120] Cases are listed in **Table 1**.

One case of an intraocular osteosarcoma causing perforation of the cornea was reported, although it is unclear if the perforation was directly from the mass or secondary to chronic exposure keratitis from the reported exophthalmia.[121]

Corneal Degeneration

Lipid keratopathy is common in parrots consistently fed high-fat diets and may develop a secondary degeneration as an inflammatory response to the lipid.[122] Corneal degeneration has been observed clinically as a postinflammatory change. Avascular corneal crystalline deposits were reported in cockatiels, parakeets, Amazon parrots, budgerigars, and finches in varying depths of the cornea, in addition to a single case of corneal dystrophy in a parakeet.[60] There is a report of bilateral corneal keratopathy demonstrated by axial stromal fibrosis in a young barred owl.[123] Two case

Table 1
Ocular surface neoplasia in birds

Location	Diagnosis	Species	Reference
Conjunctiva/sclera	Xanthoma	Blue and gold macaw	Souza et al,[106] 2009
	Presumed histiocytic sarcoma	Great horned owl	Sacre et al,[107] 1992
	Hibernoma	Goose	Murphy et al,[108] 1986
	Episclera teratoma	Turkey	Rodriguez-Ramos & Dubielzig,[66] 2015
	Squamous cell carcinoma	African gray	Rodriguez-Ramos & Dubielzig,[66] 2015
	Adenocarcinoma	Ostrich	Perrin et al,[109] 2017
Eyelid/third eyelid	Basaloid cell tumor	Parkeet	Brightman et al,[110] 1978
	Basal cell carcinoma	Conure	Kern et al,[72] 1996
	Squamous cell carcinoma	Conure	Kern et al,[72] 1996
	Epidermoid carcinoma	Red-tailed Hawk	Kern et al,[72] 1996
	Xanthoma	Budgerigar	Kern et al,[72] 1996
		Amazon	Willis & Wilkie,[53] 1999
	Mast cell tumor	Chicken	Patnaik & Mohanty,[111] 1970
	Round cell tumor	Cockatoo	Rodriguez-Ramos & Dubielzig,[66] 2015
	Chondrosarcoma	Great white heron	Spalding & Woodard,[112] 1992
Orbit	Cystadenoma	African gray	Hochleithner,[113] 1990
	Lymphosarcoma	Peafowl	Miller et al,[65] 1998
	Melanoma	African gray	Paul-Murphy et al,[114] 1985
	Lymphoma	Pigeon	Rambow et al,[115] 1981
		Peafowl	Rodriguez-Ramos & Dubielzig,[66] 2015
		Peafowl	Rodriguez-Ramos & Dubielzig,[66] 2015
	Adenoma	African gray	Simova et al,[116] 2009
	Rhabdomyosarcoma	Peregrine falcon	Freundt Coello & Schaeffer,[117] 2014
	Optic nerve glioma		Williams,[94] 1994
	Ganglioneuroma	Chicken	Rodriguez-Ramos & Dubielzig,[66] 2015
	Round cell sarcoma		Williams,[94] 1994
	Undifferentiated carcinoma	Dove	Rodriguez-Ramos & Dubielzig,[66] 2015
	Metastatic papillary cystic carcinoma	Parakeet	Rodriguez-Ramos & Dubielzig,[66] 2015
Miscellaneous	Pituitary adenoma causing exophthalmia	Cockatiel	Curtis-Velasco,[118] 1992
		Amazon	Romagnano et al,[119] 1995
		Budgerigar	Schlumberger,[120] 1954

series describe a slowly progressive lipoidal corneal degeneration in falcons that may be age related in some cases.[43,124]

MISCELLANEOUS NONINFECTIOUS DISEASES

Calcified nodules of the third eyelid conjunctiva in kestrels were an incidental finding and were untreated.[72] One case of corneal fibrosis and 1 case of crystalline deposits were identified in free-living Hummingbirds from California.[14] A survey of captive great gray owls reported chronic corneal changes in 7 out of 46 eyes.[125]

Keratoglobus of chickens has been described as a recessive sex-linked trait of females starting around 5 weeks old,[126] but has also been reported in at least 1 male chicken accidently reared with female broiler chickens, also presenting with keratoglobus at 5 weeks old.[127] In the latter report, some corneal inflammatory changes were identified histopathologically, and the underlying cause of keratoglobus was undiagnosed. A case of keratoglobus in a great horned owl was also reported.[128]

SUMMARY

In regards to avian ophthalmic disease, safe restraint, extensive history, thorough ocular and physical examinations, thorough diagnostic approach, and ability to treat are imperative to achieving a favorable outcome. Inability to treat or refractory disease may result in loss of the eye. When possible, evisceration may be preferred to enucleation. The reader is referred to reports describing surgical techniques for avian evisceration.[129–131]

REFERENCES

1. Kern TJ, Colitz CMH. Exotic animal ophthalmology. In: Gelatt KN, Gilger BC, Kern TJ, editors. Veterinary ophthalmology. 5th edition. Ames (IA): Wiley-Blackwell; 2013. p. 1750–819.
2. Williams DL, Flach E. Symblepharon with aberrant protrusion of the nictitating membrane in the snowy owl (Nyctea scandiaca). Vet Ophthalmol 2003;6(1): 11–3.
3. Kafarnik C, Fritsche J, Reese S. In vivo confocal microscopy in the normal corneas of cats, dogs and birds. Vet Ophthalmol 2007;10(4):222–30.
4. Schaeffel F, Howland HC. Corneal accommodation in chicks and pigeons. J Comp Physiol A Neuroethol Sens Neural Behav Physiol 1995;160:375–84.
5. Murphy CJ, Dubielzig RR. The gross and microscopic structure of the golden eagle (Aquila chrysaetos) eye. Prog Vet Comp Ophthalmol 1993;3:74–9.
6. Miller D, Atebara N, Stegmann R. The role of the limbal cornea in vision. Eye 1989;3:128–31.
7. Kuhn SE, Hendrix DVH, Jones MP, et al. Biometry, keratometry, and calculation of intraocular lens power for the bald eagle (Haliaeetus leucocephalus). Vet Ophthalmol 2015;18:106–12.
8. Martin GR, Katzir G. Sun shades and eye size in birds. Brain Behav Evol 2000; 56:340–4.
9. Plochocki JH, Segev T, Grow W, et al. Extraocular muscle architecture in hawks and owls. Vet Ophthalmol 2018. https://doi.org/10.1111/vop.12553.
10. Holt EK, Rosenthal FS, Shofer FS. The phenol red thread tear test in large psittaciformes. Vet Ophthalmol 2006;9:109–13.
11. Korbel R, Leitenstorfer P. Clinical estimation of lacrimal function in various bird species using a modified Schirmer tear test. J Vet Med 1996;51:171–5.

12. Falcao MS, Monteiro RV, Carvalho CM, et al. Reference values for selected ophthalmic tests of the blue-and-yellow macaw (Ara ararauna). Pesqui Vet Bras 2017;37(4):389–94.

13. Lange RR, Lima L, Przydzimirski AC, et al. Reference values for the production of the aqueous fraction of the tear film measured by the standardized endodontic absorbent paper point test in different exotic and laboratory animal species. Vet Ophthalmol 2014;17(1):41–5.

14. Moore BA, Maggs DJ, Kim S, et al. Clinical findings and normative ocular data for free-living Anna's (Calypte anna) and black-chinned (Archilochus alexandri) hummingbirds. Vet Ophthalmol 2018. https://doi.org/10.1111/vop.12560.

15. Levine J. Consensual light response in birds. Science 1955;122:690.

16. Zenoble RD, Griffith RW, Club SL. Survey of bacteriologic flora of conjunctiva and cornea in healthy psittacine birds. Am J Vet Res 1983;44:1966–7.

17. Dupont C, Carrier N, Higgins R. Bacterial and fungal flora in healthy eyes of birds of prey. Can Vet J 1994;35:699–701.

18. Beckwith-Cohen B, Horowitz I, Bdolah-Abram T, et al. Differences in ocular parameters between diurnal and nocturnal raptors. Vet Ophthalmol 2015;18(s1): 98–105.

19. Miller PE, Langenberg JA, Hartmann MT. The normal conjunctival aerobic bacterial flora of three species of captive cranes. J Zoo Wildl Med 1995;26:545–9.

20. Silvanose CD, Bailey TA, Naldo JL, et al. Bacterial flora of the conjunctiva and nasal cavity in normal and diseased captive bustards. Avian Dis 2001;45(2): 447–51.

21. Cousquer GO, Cooper JE, Cobb MA. Conjunctival flora in tawny owls (Strix aluco). Vet Rec 2010;166(21):652–4.

22. Harris MC, Schorling JJ, Herring IP, et al. Ophthalmic examination findings in a colony of screech owls (megascops asio). Vet Ophthalmol 2008;11(3):186–92.

23. Sala A, Taddei S, Santospirito D, et al. Antibiotic resistance in conjunctival and enteric bacterial flora in raptors housed in a zoological garden. Vet Med Sci 2016;2:239–45.

24. Chalmers WSK, Kewley DR. Bacterial flora of clinically normal conjunctivae in the domestic duckling. Avian Pathol 1984;14:69–74.

25. Swinger RL, Langan JN, Hamor R. Ocular bacterial flora, tear production, and intraocular pressure in a captive flock of Humboldt penguins (Spheniscus humboldti). J Zoo Wildl Med 2009;40(3):430–6.

26. Meekins JM, Stuckey JA, Carpenter JW, et al. Ophthalmic diagnostic tests and ocular findings in a flock of captive American flamingos (Phoenicopterus ruber ruber). J Avian Med Surg 2015;29(2):95–105.

27. Cheville NF, Tappe J, Ackermann M, et al. Acute fibrinopurulent blepharitis and conjunctivitis associated with Staphylococcus hyicus, Escherichia coli, and Streptococcus sp. in chickens and turkeys. Vet Pathol 1988;25:369–75.

28. Olson LD. Ophthalmia in turkeys infected with Pasteurella multocida. Avian Dis 1980;25:423–30.

29. Ley DH, Hawley DM, Geary SJ, et al. House finch (Haemorhous mexicanus) conjunctivitis, and Mycoplasma spp. isolated from North American wild birds, 1994–2015. J Wildl Dis 2016;52(3):669–73.

30. Staley M, Bonneaud C, Mcgraw KJ, et al. Detection of mycoplasma gallisepticum in house finches (Haemorhous Mexicanus) from Arizona. Avian Dis 2018; 62(1):14–7.

31. Nunoya T, Yagihashi T, Tajima M, et al. Occurrence of keratoconjunctivitis apparently caused by *Mycoplasma gallisepticum* in layer chickens. Vet Pathol 1995; 32(1):11–8.
32. Forsyth MH, Tully JG, Gorton TS, et al. *Mycoplasma sturni* sp nov from the conjunctiva of a European starling (Sturnus Vulgaris). Int J Syst Evol Microbiol 1996; 46:716–9.
33. Frasca SJ, Hinckley L, Forsyth MH, et al. Mycoplasmal conjunctivitis in a European starling. J Wildl Dis 1997;33:336–9.
34. Ley DH, Geary SH, Bekhoff JE, et al. *Mycoplasma sturni* from blue jays and northern mockingbirds with conjunctivitis in Florida. J Wildl Dis 1998;34:403–6.
35. Hawley DM, Grodio J, Frasca S Jr, et al. Experimental infection of domestic canaries (Serinus canaria domestica) with *Mycoplasma gallisepticum*: a new model system for a wildlife disease. Avian Pathol 2011;40(3):321–7.
36. Mashima TY, Ley DH, Stoskopf MK, et al. Evaluation of treatment of conjunctivitis associated with *Mycoplasma gallisepticum* in house finches (Carpodacus mexicanus). J Avian Med Surg 1997;1(1):20–4.
37. Maddux RL, Chengappa MM, McLaughlin BG. Isolation of *Actinobacillus suis* from a Canada goose (Branta canadensis). J Wildl Dis 1987;23(3):483–4.
38. Hacking MA, Sileo L. Isolation of a hemolytic Actinobacillus from waterfowl. J Wildl Dis 1977;13(1):69–73.
39. Hvenegaard AP, Safatle A, Guimarães MB, et al. Retrospective study of ocular disorders in Amazon parrots. Pesqui Vet Bras 2009;29(12):979–84.
40. Shimakura S, Sawa H, Yamashita T, et al. An outbreak of ocular disease caused by staphylococcal infection in amazon parrot (Amazona aestiva) imported into Japan. Jpn J Vet Sci 1981;43(2):273–5.
41. Pocknell AM, Miller BJ, Neufeld JL, et al. Conjunctival mycobacteriosis in two emus (Dromaius novaehollandiae). Vet Pathol 1996;33(3):346–8.
42. Stanz KM, Miller PE, Cooley AJ, et al. Mycobacterial keratitis in a parrot. J Am Vet Med Assoc 1995;206:1177–80.
43. Kern TJ, editor. Disorders of the special senses. Philadelphia: W.B. Saunders; 1997.
44. Miller PE, Langenberg JA, Baeten LA, et al. Pseudomonas aeruginosa-associated corneal ulcers in captive cranes. J Zoo Wildl Med 1994;1:449–54.
45. Surman PG, Schultz DJ, Tham VL. Keratoconjunctivitis and chlamydiosis in cage birds. Aust Vet J 1974;50(8):356–62.
46. Farmer H, Chalmers WS, Woolcock PR. *Chlamydia psittaci* isolated from the eyes of domestic ducks (Anas platyrhynchos) with conjunctivitis and rhinitis. Vet Rec 1982;110(3):59.
47. Saroglu M, Yucel R, Aktas M. Granulomatous conjunctivitis in an ostrich. Vet Ophthalmol 2003;6(4):337–9.
48. Graham CL. Poxvirus infection in a spectacled Amazon parrot (Amazona albifrons). Avian Dis 1978;22(2):340–3.
49. McDonald SE, Lowenstine LJ, Ardans AA. Avian pox in blue-fronted Amazon parrots. J Am Vet Med Assoc 1981;179(11):1218–22.
50. Johnson BJ, Castro AE. Canary pox causing high mortality in an aviary. J Am Vet Med Assoc 1986;189(10):1345–7.
51. Docherty DE, Long RI, Flickinger EL, et al. Isolation of poxvirus from debilitating cutaneous lesions on four immature grackles (Quiscalus sp). Avian Dis 1991;35:244–7.
52. Docherty DE, Long RI. Isolation of a poxvirus from a house finch, Carpodacus mexicanus (Müller). J Wildl Dis 1986;22(3):420–2.

53. Willis AM, Wilkie DA. Avian ophthalmology, part 2: review of ophthalmic diseases. J Avian Med Surg 1999;13(4):245–51.

54. Tompkins EM, Anderson DJ, Pabilonia KL, et al. Avian pox discovered in the critically endangered waved albatross (Phoebastria irrorata) from the galápagos islands, ecuador. J Wildl Dis 2017;53(4):891–5.

55. Boosinger TR, Winterfield RW, Feldman DS, et al. Psittacine pox virus: virus isolation and identification, transmission, and cross-challenge studies in parrots and chickens. Avian Dis 1982;26(2):437–44.

56. Abrams GA, Paul-Murphy J, Murphy CJ. Conjunctivitis in birds. Vet Clin North Am Exot Anim Pract 2002;5(2):287–309.

57. Pandiri AK, Cortes AL, Lee LF, et al. Marek's disease virus infection in the eye: chronological study of the lesions, virus replication, and vaccine-induced protection. Avian Dis 2008;52(4):572–80.

58. Gleeson MD, Moore BA, Edwards SG, et al. A novel herpesvirus associated with chronic superficial keratitis and proliferative conjunctivitis in a great horned owl (Bubo virginanus). Vet Ophthalmol 2018. https://doi.org/10.1111/vop.12570.

59. Susta L, Miller PJ, Afonso CL, et al. Pathogenicity evaluation of different Newcastle disease virus chimeras in 4-week-old chickens. Trop Anim Health Prod 2010;42(8):1785–95.

60. Tsai SS, Park JH, Hirai K, et al. Eye lesions in pet birds. Avian Pathol 1993;22: 95–112.

61. Jacobson ER, Mladinich CR, Clubb S, et al. Papilloma-like virus infection in an African gray parrot. J Am Vet Med Assoc 1983;193:1307–8.

62. Desmidt M, Ducatelle R, Uyttebroek E, et al. Cytomegalovirus-like conjunctivitis in Australian finches. J Assoc Avian Vet 1991;5:132–6.

63. Bui VN, Ogawa H, Ngo LH, et al. H5N1 highly pathogenic avian influenza virus isolated from conjunctiva of a whooper swan with neurological signs. Arch Virol 2013;158:451–5.

64. Pauli AM, Cruz-Martinez LA, Ponder JB, et al. Ophthalmologic and oculopathologic findings in red-tailed hawks and Cooper's hawks with naturally acquired West Nile virus infection. J Am Vet Med Assoc 2007;231:1240–8.

65. Miller PE, Paul-Murphy J, Sullivan R, et al. Orbital lymphosarcoma associated with reticuloendotheliosis virus in a peafowl. J Am Vet Med Assoc 1998; 213(3):377–80.

66. Rodriguez-Ramos Fernández J, Dubielzig RR. Ocular and eyelid neoplasia in birds: 15 cases (1982–2011). Vet Ophthalmol 2015;18(s1):113–8.

67. Kennedy FA, Buggage RR, Ajello L. Rhinosporidiosis: a description of an unprecedented outbreak in captive swans (Cygnus spp.) and a proposal for revision of the ontogenic nomenclature of Rhinosporidium seeberi. J Med Vet Mycol 1995;33(3):157–65.

68. McCowan C, Bibby S, Scott PC. Mycotic keratitis due to Scedosporium apiospermum in layer pullets. Vet Ophthalmol 2014;17(1):63–6.

69. Abrams GA, Paul-Murphy J, Ramer JC, et al. Aspergillus blepharitis and dermatitis in a peregrine falcon-gyrfalcon hybrid (Falco peregrinus× Falco rusticolus). J Avian Med Surg 2001;15(2):114–20.

70. Hoppes S, Gurfield N, Flammer K, et al. Mycotic keratitis in a blue-fronted amazon parrot (Amazona aestive). J Avian Med Surg 2000;14(3):185–9.

71. Sadar MJ, Sanchez-Migallon G, Burton AG, et al. Mycotic keratitis in a khaki campbell duck (Anas platyrhynchos domesticus). J Avian Med Surg 2014; 28(4):322–9.

72. Kern TJ, Paul-Murphy J, Murphy CJ, et al. Disorders of the third eyelid in birds: 17 cases. J Avian Med Surg 1996;10(1):12–8.

73. Crispin SM, Barnett KC. Ocular candidiasis in ornamental ducks. Avian Pathol 1978;7(1):49–59.

74. Tsai SS, Park JH, Hirai K, et al. Aspergillosis and candidiasis in psittacine and passeriform birds with particular reference to nasal lesions. Avian Pathol 1992;21(4):699–709.

75. Mustaffa-Babjee AH. Specific and non-specific conditions affecting avian eyes. Vet Bull 1969;39(10):681–7.

76. Verocai GG, Lopes LN, Burlini L, et al. Occurrence of *Philophthalmus gralli* (Trematoda: philophthalmidae) in farmed ostriches in Brazil. Trop Anim Health Prod 2009;41:1241–2.

77. Church ML, Barrett PM, Swenson J, et al. Outbreak of *Philophthalmus grallis* in four greater rheas (Rhea americana). Vet Ophthalmol 2013;16(1):65–72.

78. Nollen PM, Murray HD. Philophthalmus gralli: identification, growth characteristics, and treatment of an oriental eyefluke of birds introduced into the continental United States. J Parasitol 1978;64(1):178–80.

79. Rodriguez-Tovar LE, Casas-Martinez A, Ramirez-Romero R, et al. First report of *Oxyspirura* sp from a captive fulvous owl. J Parasitol 2008;94(6):1430–1.

80. Bruno A, Fedynich AM, Smith-Herron A, et al. Pathological response of northern bobwhites to *Oxyspirura petrowi* infections. J Parasitol 2015;101(3):364–8.

81. Dunham NR, Soliz LA, Brightman A, et al. Live eyeworm (*Oxyspirura petrowi*) extraction, in vitro culture, and transfer for experimental studies. J Parasitol 2015;101(1):98–101.

82. Dunham NR, Peper ST, Baxter CE, et al. The parasitic eye worm *Oxyspirura petrowi* as a possible cause of decline in the threatened lesser prairie-chicken (Tympanuchus pallidicinctus). PLoS One 2014;9(9):e108244.

83. Suedmeyer WK, Smith T, Moore C, et al. *Ceratospira inglisi* ocular infestation in a Wompoo fruit-dove (Ptilinopus magnificus). J Avian Med Surg 1999;13(4): 261–4.

84. Brooks DE, Greiner EC, Walsh MT. Conjunctivitis caused by Thelazia sp in a Senegal parrot. J Am Vet Med Assoc 1983;183(11):1305–6.

85. Murata K, Asakawa M. First report of Thelazia sp. from a captive Oriental white stork (Ciconia boyciana) in Japan. J Vet Med Sci 1999;61(1):93–5.

86. De Jong AC. *Plasmodium dissanaikei* n sp a new avian malaria parasite from the rose-ringed parakeet of Ceylon, Psittacula krameri manillensis. Ceylon Journal of Med Science 1971;20:41–5.

87. Randall CJ. Conjunctivitis in pheasants associated with cryptosporidial infection. Vet Rec 1986;118:211–2.

88. Mason RW. Conjunctival cryptosporidiosis in a duck. Avian Dis 1986;30(3): 598–600.

89. Mason RW, Hartley WJ. Respiratory cryptosporidiosis in a peacock chick. Avian Dis 1980;24(3):771–6.

90. Molina-Lopez RA, Ramis A, Martín-Vázquez S, et al. Cryptosporidium baileyi infection associated with an outbreak of ocular and respiratory disease in otus owls (Otus scops) in a rehabilitation centre. Avian Pathol 2010;39(3):171–6.

91. Phalen DN, Logan KS, Snowden KF. Encephalitozoon hellem infection as the cause of a unilateral chronic keratoconjunctivitis in an umbrella cockatoo (Cacatua alba). Vet Ophthalmol 2006;9(1):59–63.

92. Karakavuk M, Aykur M, Sahar EA, et al. First time identification of acanthamoeba genotypes in the cornea samples of wild birds. Is acanthamoeba keratitis making the predatory birds a target. Exp Parasitol 2017;183:137–42.
93. Kern TJ, Murphy CJ, Heck WR. Partial upper eyelid agenesis in a Peregrine falcon. J Am Vet Med Assoc 1985;187(11):1207.
94. Williams D. Ophthalmology. In: Richie BW, Harrison CJ, editors. Avian medicine: principles and practice. Lake Worth (FL): Wingers Publishing; 1994. p. 673–94.
95. Busch TJ. Letter to the editor: bilateral dermoids in a goose. N Z Vet J 1985;33: 189–90.
96. Leber AC, Burge T. A dermoid of the eye in a blue-fronted Amazon parrot (Amazona aestiva). Vet Ophthalmol 1999;2:133–5.
97. O'Connell KM, Michau TM, Stine JM, et al. Ophthalmic diagnostic testing and examination findings in a colony of captive brown pelicans (Pelecanus occidentalis). Vet Ophthalmol 2017;20(3):196–204.
98. Freeman KS, Fiorello C, Murray M. Comparison of anterior segment health in wild and captive common murres. Vet Ophthalmol 2018;21(2):174–81.
99. Seruca C, Molina-Lopez R, Pena T, et al. Ocular consequences of blunt trauma in two species of nocturnal raptors (Athene noctua and Octus scops). Vet Ophthalmol 2012;15(4):236–44.
100. Murphy CJ, Kern TJ, McKeever K, et al. Ocular lesions in free-living raptors. J Am Vet Med Assoc 1982;181:1302–4.
101. Moore BA, Teixeira LBC, Sponsel WE, et al. The consequences of avian ocular trauma: histopathological evidence and implications of acute and chronic disease. Vet Ophthalmol 2017;20(6):496–504.
102. Gionfriddo JR, Powell CC. Primary closure of the corneas of two great horned owls after resection of nonhealing ulcers. Vet Ophthalmol 2006;9(4):251–4.
103. Andrew SE, Clippinger TL, Brooks DE, et al. Penetrating keratoplasty for treatment of corneal protrusion in a great horned owl (Bubo virginianus). Vet Ophthalmol 2002;5(3):202–5.
104. Lynch GL, Scagliotti RH, Hoffman A, et al. Penetrating keratoplasty in a California Brown Pelican. Vet Ophthalmol 2007;10(4):254–61.
105. Raidal SR. Staphylococcal dermatitis in quail with parakeratotic hyperkeratotic dermatosis suggestive of pantothenic acid deficiency. Avian Dis 1994;24: 579–83.
106. Souza MJ, Johnstone-McLean NS, Ward D, et al. Conjunctival xanthoma in a blue and gold macaw (Ara Ararauna). Vet Ophthalmol 2009;12(1):53–5.
107. Sacre BJ, Oppenheim YC, Steinberg H, et al. Presumptive histiocytic sarcoma in a great horned owl (Bubo virginianus). J Zoo Wildl Med 1992;23(1):113–21.
108. Murphy CJ, Bellhorn RW, Buyukmihci N. Subconjunctival hibernoma in a goose. J Am Vet Med Assoc 1986;189(9):1109–10.
109. Perrin KL, Bertelsen MF, Bartholin H, et al. Conjunctival mucinous adenocarcinoma in an ostrich (Struthio camelus). Vet Ophthalmol 2017;20(6):547–50.
110. Brightman AH, Burke TJ. Eyelid tumor in a parakeet. Mod Vet Pract 1978;59(9): 683.
111. Patnaik GM, Mohanty D. A case of avian mastocytoma. Indian Vet J 1970;47: 298–300.
112. Spalding MG, Woodard JC. Chondrosarcoma in a wild great white heron from southern Florida. J Wildl Dis 1992;28(1):151–3.
113. Hochleithner M. Cystadenoma in an African grey parrot (Psittacus erithacus). J Assoc Avian Veterinarians 1990;4:163–6.

114. Paul-Murphy J, Lowenstine L, Turrel JM, et al. Malignant lymphoreticular neoplasm in an African gray parrot. J Am Vet Med Assoc 1985;187(11):1216–7.
115. Rambow VJ, Murphy JC, Fox JG. Malignant lymphoma in a pigeon. J Am Vet Med Assoc 1981;179(11):1266–8.
116. Simova-Curd S, Richter M, Hauser B, et al. Surgical removal of a retrobulbar adenoma in an African grey parrot (Psittacus erithacus). J Avian Med Surg 2009; 23(1):24–8.
117. Freundt Coello MJ, Schaeffer LS. Retrobulbar rhabdomyosarcoma in a neotropical peregrine falcon (Falco peregrinus cassini). Vet Ophthalmol 2014;17(1): 73–5.
118. Curtis-Velasco M. Pituitary adenoma in a cockatiel (Nymphicus hollandicus). J Assoc Avian Veterinarians 1992;6:21–2.
119. Romagnano A, Mashima TY, Barnes HJ, et al. Pituitary adenoma in an amazon parrot. J Avian Med Surg 1995;9(4):263–70.
120. Schlumberger HG. Neoplasia in the parakeet. I. Spontaneous chromophobe pituitary tumors. Cancer Res 1954;14:237–45.
121. Fordham M, Rosenthal K, Durham A, et al. Intraocular osteosarcoma in an umbrella cockatoo (cacatua alba). Vet Ophthalmol 2010;13:103–8.
122. Doneley B. Disorders of the eye. In: Doneley B, editor. Avian medicine and surgery in practice: companion and aviary birds. 2nd edition. Boca Raton (FL): CRC Press; 2016. p. 197–203.
123. Murphy CJ, Kern TJ, MacCoy DM. Bilateral keratopathy in a barred owl. J Am Vet Med Assoc 1982;179(11):1271–3.
124. Moore BA, Paul-Murphy JR, Adamson KL, et al. Lipoidal corneal degeneration in aged falcons. Vet Ophthalmol 2018;21(4):332–8.
125. Wills S, Pinard C, Nykamp S, et al. Ophthalmic reference values and lesions in two captive populations of northern owls: great grey owls (Strix nebulosa) and snowy owls (Bubo scandiacus). J Zoo Wildl Med 2016;47(1):244–55.
126. Bitgood JJ, Whitley RD. Pop eye: an inherited Z-linked keratoglobus in the chicken. J Hered 1986;77:123–5.
127. Landman WJM, Boeve MH, Dwars RM, et al. Keratoglobus lesions in the eyes of rearing broiler breeders. Avian Pathol 1998;27(3):256–62.
128. Lau RK, Moresco A, Woods SJ, et al. Presumptive keratoglobus in a great horned owl (Bubo virginianus). Vet Ophthalmol 2017;20(6):560–7.
129. Christen C, Richter M, Fischer I, et al. Unilateral evisceration of an eye following cornea and lens perforation in a sulfur-crested cockatoo (Cacatua galerita). Schweiz Arch Tierheilkd 2006;148(11):615–9.
130. Murray M, Pizzirani S, Tseng F. A technique for evisceration as an alternative to enucleation in birds of prey: 19 cases. J Avian Med Surg 2013;27(2):120–7.
131. Dees DD, Knollinger AM, MacLaren NE. Modified evisceration technique in a golden eagle (Aquila chrysaetos). Vet Ophthalmol 2011;14(5):341–4.

Ocular Surface Disease in New World Camelids

Sarah L. Czerwinski, DVM, DACVO

KEYWORDS

- Camelid • Alpaca • Llama • Ocular surface • Cornea • Conjunctiva • Tears

KEY POINTS

- The large, prominent globes of camelids predispose them to corneal trauma. Ocular disease is mostly traumatic; some inherited and congenital abnormalities have been reported.
- Camelids are predisposed to developing profound corneal edema due to suspected corneal endothelial cell fragility, which may present additional challenges in managing corneal disease.
- Conditions affecting the ocular surface, including conjunctivitis, keratoconjunctivitis, and ulcerative keratitis should be treated with broad spectrum topical antimicrobial medication. Culture and cytology may provide further information to guide therapy.

INTRODUCTION

The family, Camelidae is made up of 3 genera: *Camelus*, *Lama*, and *Vicugna*. Old World camelids include the dromedary camel (*Camelus dromedarius*) and the Bactrian camel (*Camelus bactrianus*). The 4 species comprising the New World camelids include the llama (*Lama glama*) and guacano (*Lama guanicoe*), belonging to the genus *Lama*, the alpaca (*Vicugna pacos*), which has been reclassified into the genus *Vicugna* based on new genetic information, and the vicugna (*Vicugna vicugna*), also in the genus *Vicugna*.[1] This article focuses on the New World camelids, the alpaca and llama.

Alpacas and llamas have become increasingly popular in North America. They are kept for their fiber, as pets, as companions for other animals, and even as therapy animals. Currently there are 191,460 registered alpacas in the United States and 13,476 in Canada.[2] There are fewer registered llamas in North America: 30,464 in the United States and 1122 in Canada.[3] These numbers include only registered animals; actual numbers can be expected to be much higher. It is likely that the many veterinarians, both small animal and large animal alike, will encounter a camelid as a patient.

Ocular surface disease, often related to trauma, is common in camelids.[4] Similar to horses, this is likely related to their prominent globes and their environment. Inherited and congenital diseases also have been reported.[5,6]

Disclosure Statement: No disclosures.
Department of Small Animal Medicine and Surgery, University of Georgia Veterinary Teaching Hospital, 2200 College Station Road, Athens, GA 30602, USA
E-mail address: Sarah.Czerwinski@uga.edu

The ophthalmic examination is best conducted in a quiet, dark environment, using a bright light source, such as a transilluminator. Depending on how much restraint is required, they can be examined while standing in stocks or a stall, or in a cushed position in a stall. Although sedation is usually not required, butorphanol at a reported dose of 0.02 to 0.04 mg/kg can help to stabilize the head when necessary, although doses as high as 0.05–0.1 mg/kg IM or IV may be used.[7]

ANATOMY AND PHYSIOLOGY

New World camelids have very large globes relative to their skull and body size. Lateral placement on the skull allows for immense peripheral vision. Their eyelids hug the globe tightly and are lined by long cilia that shield the cornea. Long vibrissae provide tactile sensation (**Figs. 1** and **2**).

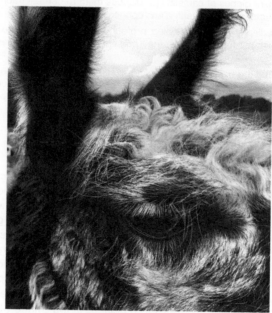

Fig. 1. External ocular anatomy of an adult llama (Lama glama).

Precorneal Tear Film

The precorneal tear film is an important part of the ocular defense system. In addition to aiding in removal of debris from the ocular surface in conjunction with the eyelids, it lubricates the corneal and conjunctival surface to prevent desiccation, and contains enzymes, proteins, and immunoglobulins as part of the ocular defense system against pathogens.

The aqueous portion of the tear film is produced by the lacrimal gland. Because camelids do not have lipid-producing meibomian glands lining their eyelid margin, it is suspected that the lipid portion of the tear film is produced by sebaceous glands located on the nictitans and caruncle.[8] The upper eyelid of the 1-humped camel has mucous glands that open onto the conjunctival surface near the eyelid margin, but such a structure has not been identified in llamas or alpacas.[9]

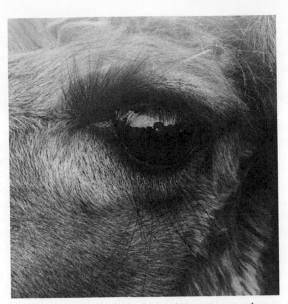

Fig. 2. External ocular anatomy of an adult alpaca (Vicugna pacos).

Tear production is quantified in mm/min using a Schirmer tear test (STT) strip placed in the lower eyelid. In normal llamas, the STT I, a measure of the basal and reflex tear production, and STT II, the basal tear production alone, were 17.3 ± 1.1 mm/min (range 15–19 mm/min) and 15.4 ± 1.7 mm/min (range 12.5–17.5 mm/min), respectively.[10] The STT I in normal alpacas was 20.88 ± 4.04 mm/min.[11]

The composition of llama tear film has been extensively evaluated to determine species differences that may affect susceptibility to infectious ocular surface disease. Llama tears have a pH of 8.05 ± 0.01, similar to that of cattle but a significantly higher protein concentration 7.50 ± 1.9 mg/mL.[12] Tears of healthy llamas were found to contain substances contributing to the ocular defense system, including the chelating proteins lactoferrin, ceruloplasmin, and transferrin, the anticollagenases α-1 antitrypsin, and α-2 macroglobulin, and immunoglobulin (Ig)A.[12] Llamas were shown to have higher tear levels of lysozyme than sheep and bovines, using 2 different assays.[13] Although not a species of focus of this article, it is interesting to note that a study examining the protein composition of camel tears identified large quantities of human vitelline membrane outer layer protein 1 (VMO1),[14] a protein that was later shown to interact with lysozyme and increase stability of the tear film.[15] Interestingly, tear levels of VMO1 vary seasonally, with higher levels present in summer versus winter.[16] Although the presence of this protein has not been evaluated in New World camelids to the author's knowledge, it further suggests the possibility of species-specific adaptations of the ocular surface that may explain differences in susceptibility to disease.

The tears drain into the upper and lower nasolacrimal puncta, 2 small openings located 4 to 6 mm from the medial canthus. The puncta connect to the dorsal and ventral canaliculi, which empty into a single lacrimal sac. The sac connects to the nasolacrimal duct, which courses through the maxilla and terminates in the ventral nasal vestibule. In the adult llama, the duct is 11 to 15 cm long with a diameter of 2 to 4 mm.[17]

Conjunctiva

The conjunctiva is essentially a sheet of connective tissue and overlying epithelium that covers the sclera from the limbus, forms the fornix, and covers the bulbar surface of the upper and lower eyelids, as well as the nictitans. In camelids, the conjunctiva and sclera are often darkly pigmented, especially the 2-mm to 3-mm area immediately adjacent to the limbus, which is thought to have a protective effect against UV light.[8]

The conjunctiva is a critical part of the mucosal immune system. Commensal organisms normally inhabit the conjunctiva, and several species of aerobic bacteria and fungi have been isolated from the conjunctival sacs of healthy camelids. Across several studies that have been performed in New World camelids, *Staphylococcus* spp are most commonly isolated.[18,19] Potentially pathogenic bacteria isolated from the conjunctival sac of normal alpacas, llamas, and guanacos include *Streptomyces*, *Pasteurella*, *Corynebacterium*, and several species of *Pseudomonas*. *Mycoplasma* has not been identified in the conjunctiva of normal camelids.[18] Many genera of fungi have been isolated, *Aspergillus* sp most commonly, and are assumed to be from normal exposure in the environment.[20]

Moraxella ovis and *Moraxella catarrhalis* have been isolated from the conjunctival sac of normal Huacaya alpacas in Belgium. These isolates were significantly more likely to be found in younger animals.[19] Although *Moraxella* spp is the causative agent of infectious bovine keratoconjunctivitis, there are few reports of this bacteria causing disease in camelids.[21]

Cornea

The cornea of the New World camelid is oval in shape, with a mean horizontal diameter that is greater than the vertical diameter. In both species, the cornea is approximately 0.6-mm thick. The cornea was found to be significantly thinner in young llamas, but not alpacas.[22] (**Table 1**) Corneal sensitivity, measured using a Cochet-Bonnet anesthesiometer, was determined to be greatest in the central cornea in alpacas. Crias have increased corneal sensitivity compared with adults.[23]

The corneal endothelium is essential for maintaining relative stromal dehydration. The corneal endothelial cell density is similar in alpacas and llamas, but decreased with age only in the llama.[22] In both species, the endothelial cells were often heterogeneous, which may indicate endothelial cell fragility and explain why New World camelids are susceptible to developing profound corneal edema.[22]

Table 1 Various corneal measurements		
Parameter	Alpaca	Llama
Mean corneal diameter Horizontal	30.2 ± 0.2 mm	28.2 ± 0.4 mm
Mean corneal diameter Vertical	22.2 ± 0.2 mm	22.5 ± 0.3 mm
Mean corneal thickness	595 ± 9 μm	608 ± 5 μm
Endothelial cell density	2275 ± 90 cells/mm^2	2669 ± 56 cells/mm^2

Data from Andrew SE, Ramsey DT, Hauptman JG, et al. Density of corneal endothelial cells and corneal thickness in eyes of euthanatized horses. Am J Vet Res 2001;62(4):479–82. ISSN 0002-9045. Available at: http://www.ncbi.nlm.nih.gov/pubmed/11327451.

DISEASES
Congenital/Inherited

There are few reports of congenital and inherited disease in New World camelids. There is a report of a conjunctival cyst in the ventrotemporal bulbar conjunctiva of a cria, suspected to be congenital.[24] Conjunctival dermoids have been reported in llamas.[4] As in other species, excision is expected to be curative.

Atresia of the nasolacrimal system has been reported in New World camelids, although it is more common in alpacas than llamas.[8] The nasolacrimal duct and/or the puncta, both proximal and distal, may be affected. Signs of nasolacrimal atresia include epiphora, with the periocular area appearing wet with tears. Dacryocystitis may occur secondarily, producing mucopurulent discharge. Diagnosis depends on the location of the atresia and may include examination (absence of visible puncta in the eyelid or nares), inability to lavage the duct with sterile saline or eyewash, and contrast dacryocystorrhinography to diagnose the location of the atresia. Four young alpacas with nasal punctal atresia were successfully treated by incision of the imperforate tissue and placement of a stent.[25] A 2-month-old alpaca with bilateral atresia of the middle of the duct was treated successfully by creation of new outflow tracts from the conjunctiva, with a conjunctivorhinostomy in one eye and a conjunctivomaxillosinusotomy in the other.[26]

Corneal dystrophy, manifesting as a nonprogressive anterior stromal crystalline opacity, has been reported in the alpaca,[6] in addition to other nonpublished reports.[8]

Acquired

Dacryocystitis

Dacryocystitis, inflammation of the lacrimal sac, often presents with chronic mucopurulent ocular discharge, conjunctival hyperemia, and sometimes blepharospasm.[8] As discussed previously, it can be secondary to a congenital atresia, or acquired, as the large nasal puncta are an easy entry for foreign bodies such as grass awns, that can become trapped within the lacrimal sac causing persistent inflammation.

Diagnosis of dacryocystitis Dacryocystitis is diagnosed by clinical signs of nasolacrimal duct obstruction, mainly epiphora and mucopurulent ocular discharge. Visualization of conjunctival and nasal puncta and successful nasolacrimal lavage helps to differentiate primary dacryocystitis from dacryocystitis secondary to nasolacrimal duct atresia.

Therapy for dacryocystitis Therapy for dacryocystitis involves retrograde and/or normograde nasolacrimal lavage with sterile saline or eyewash to remove foreign bodies, debris, and infectious agents from the duct. Often this requires sedation or general anesthesia, depending on the patient's temperament. Topical antibiotics alone are unlikely to result in clinical resolution.[8]

Conjunctivitis

Clinical signs of conjunctivitis include conjunctival hyperemia, blepharospasm, epiphora, and chemosis.[4] An older study of llamas with conjunctival disease reported that in 10% of cases there was no detectable cause.[4]

Bacterial conjunctivitis There are a few reports of infectious conjunctivitis in camelids, although it seems relatively uncommon. Bacterial conjunctivitis was identified as a cause of conjunctivitis in some cases in the 1997 study.[4] Clinical signs in these cases were severe, including mucopurulent discharge, hyperemia, and blepharospasm.[8] Gionfriddo reported 5 unpublished cases in which pathogenic bacterial organisms were cultured from the lower conjunctival fornix and was suspected to be the causative agent.[8] Other organisms, such as *Staphylococcus aureus* and chlamydiae, have been identified in the conjunctiva.[8,27] Although not affecting a New World camelid, there is a report of an outbreak of keratoconjunctivitis in a dromedary cattle herd in Spain where a biovar of *Moraxella canis* was isolated.[21]

Parasitic conjunctivitis Conjunctivitis in camelids also can be caused by the parasite *Thelazia californiensis*, transmitted between animals by flies. The nematode larvae cause physical irritation in the conjunctival sac, leading to clinical signs of epiphora, conjunctival hyperemia, chemosis, and sometimes corneal ulceration from self-trauma.[8]

There is a single unpublished report of the uveitis and associated conjunctivitis due to the protozoa, *Toxoplasma gondii*, which was definitively diagnosed by detection of rising antibody levels in the vitreous humor.[8]

Conjunctivitis secondary to foreign bodies Following an outbreak of blepharospasm and mucopurulent ocular discharge in 21 alpacas, 6 animals were diagnosed with conjunctivitis, and 5 animals were diagnosed with temporal ulcerative keratitis, edema, and vascularization.[28] Seven plant foreign bodies were found in 5 animals. They were removed with topical anesthesia and recovery was uneventful.

Diagnosis of conjunctivitis Primary conjunctivitis is diagnosed based on clinical signs, and the absence of uveitis and keratitis. In addition to a complete ophthalmic examination, including thorough evaluation of the conjunctival fornices for any potential foreign bodies, recommended diagnostic tests include cytology of conjunctival scraping and bacterial and fungal culture and sensitivity. It is important to carefully inspect the eyelids for foreign bodies in cases of temporally located corneal ulcers.

Therapy for conjunctivitis Therapy for conjunctivitis depends on the underlying cause. For bacterial conjunctivitis, topical antimicrobials should be broad-spectrum, and may need to be modified based on response to treatment and culture and sensitivity results.

If nematode larvae are identified, they should be manually removed following topical anesthesia of the ocular surface with proparacaine or tetracaine. Small cilia forceps, sterile cotton-tipped applicators, and irrigation with sterile saline or eyewash in a 3-mL to 6-mL syringe with a 25-g needle broken off at the hub are useful tools to remove these larvae, which often hide beneath the third eyelid. Cotton-tipped applicators can be used to atraumatically "sweep" the dorsal and ventral conjunctival fornices. Diligent fly control is important to prevent reinfection.

CORNEAL DISEASE

Clinical signs of keratitis may be subtle or severe, depending on whether it is ulcerative or nonulcerative, how much of the cornea is affected, and the amount of associated uveitis that is present. Signs may include blepharospasm, epiphora, mucopurulent ocular discharge, conjunctivitis, chemosis, scleral injection, corneal vascularization, pigmentation, cellular infiltrate, and corneal edema.

Corneal disease is common in camelids. It was reported as the most common disease affecting the camelid eye: 41% of llamas in one study.[4] Surveys of apparently normal alpacas without overt signs of ocular disease revealed corneal fibrosis indicating previous corneal ulceration or trauma.[6,29] The cornea is prone to developing profound corneal edema associated with corneal ulcerations, trauma, or uveitis. The reason for this is suspected to be the heterogeneity of the endothelial cells in the normal camelids, possibility indicating increased susceptibility of these cells to damage.[22]

Trauma: The camelid globe is prominent, predisposing them to corneal trauma and ulceration.

Foreign bodies: Conjunctival plant foreign body was the cause of an outbreak of conjunctivitis and ulcerative keratitis in a herd of alpacas.[28] The conjunctival fornices should be thoroughly evaluated for the presence of foreign bodies in cases of ulcerative and nonulcerative keratitis.

Indolent corneal ulcers/spontaneous chronic corneal epithelial defects (SCCEDs): Corneal ulcers that fail to heal in the expected amount of time, are not infected, without a clinically detectable underlying cause, and contain a loose rim of corneal epithelium are considered indolent. Although the cause of indolent corneal ulcers in camelids is unknown, one report in a llama suggested a similar disease as is seen in dogs, and was treated successfully with a grid keratotomy.[30]

Bacterial and Fungal Keratitis

There is a single case of *Moraxella liquefaciens* isolated from a corneal ulcer in a llama.[27] As previously discussed in the conjunctiva section, *M canis* was identified in an outbreak of keratoconjunctivitis in camels, but has not been identified as a pathogen in New World camelids,[21]

Fungal keratitis in 11 alpacas presented as stromal corneal ulceration, corneal perforation, deep stromal abscess, and nonulcerative keratitis.[31] *Aspergillus* and *Fusarium* spp were most commonly identified. One case was diagnosed with a corneal ulcer and plant foreign body 5 weeks before presentation. Deep stromal abscess in camelids is similar to the disease in horses, usually following microtrauma, which seeds bacterial or fungal organisms in the cornea. When the overlying epithelium heals, the organisms are trapped within the corneal stroma (**Fig. 3**). Unlike in horses, corneal abscesses in camelids seem to heal rapidly with medical therapy.[8]

A llama with multifocal corneal abscesses, later were diagnosed on histopathology as *Coccidioides posadasii*, which was disseminated.[32]

For ulcerative keratitis, treatment is ideally based on cytology results. Broad-spectrum antibiotics should be initiated and modified based on bacterial susceptibility results. Depending on geographic location, it may be prudent to start topical antifungal therapy prophylactically and submit a fungal culture, even if fungi is not present on cytology.

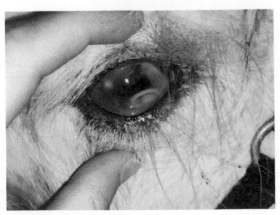

Fig. 3. The right eye of an alpaca with a large stromal abscess (axial horizontal, creamy area of infiltrate) and focal circular stromal abscess in the dorsotemporal cornea. (*Courtesy of* K. Bedard.)

Viral Keratitis

Dendritic, superficial corneal ulceration, similar to is observed with Feline Herpesvirus-1 in cats, have been reported. Although the diagnosis was not confirmed with testing, response to treatment with topical antiviral medication cidofovir suggested a viral etiology.[8]

Inclusion Cysts

Epithelial inclusion cysts were diagnosed in a mature female llama, thought to have occurred secondary to trauma or due a corneal biopsy that was obtained to diagnose an SCCED. Treatment with a keratectomy and conjunctival advancement flap was successful.[33]

Calcific Degeneration

Calcific degeneration appears as a lacey, refractile epithelial opacity, ulcerative or nonulcerative corneal opacity. Bilateral calcific band keratopathy, calcific degeneration occurring in the interpalpebral fissure, was confirmed histologically in a 4-year-old alpaca euthanized for systemic disease. The condition was nonulcerative and there was no identifiable underlying cause.[34]

Lipid Keratopathy

Lipid keratopathy, appearing as bilateral refractile corneal opacity, was described in a hypercholesterolemic alpaca.[35]

Papilloma

There is a report of a camel with a corneal mass, diagnosed as a corneal papilloma. The clinical signs of keratoconjunctivitis resolved following excisional keratectomy.[36]

Diagnosis of keratitis

Keratitis is diagnosed based on clinical signs. In addition to a complete ophthalmic examination, including thorough evaluation of the conjunctival fornices for any potential foreign bodies, recommended diagnostic tests for ulcerative lesions include cytology and bacterial and fungal culture and sensitivity. It is important to carefully inspect the eyelids for foreign bodies in cases of temporally located corneal ulcers.

In cases of complicated corneal ulcerations (those that are deep, infected, or melting), and those that fail to heal within the expected 5-day to 7-day period, corneal cytology should be performed following the application of topical anesthesia with proparacaine or tetracaine. If signs of infection are present, including white or yellow infiltrate, keratomalacia (melting), or more than mild uveitis, or there are organisms present on cytology, it is prudent to submit corneal swab samples of the ulcer for aerobic bacterial culture and sensitivity. In cases in which fungal organisms are identified on cytology, or in regions in which fungal disease is prevalent, such as the southeastern United States, submitting corneal swab samples for fungal culture and susceptibility also should be considered.

Therapy for keratitis

For cases of ulcerative keratitis, broad-spectrum antimicrobials should be initiated every 6 hours for prophylaxis of infection for superficial, noninfected ulcers, and based on cytology results for complicated ulcers. The antimicrobials should be modified where necessary based on sensitivity and susceptibility results in addition to response to treatment.

Perforated ulcers and deep ulcers at risk for perforation can be treated with keratectomy and conjunctival graft placement to stabilize the cornea and provide a blood supply necessary for healing. There is a report of an adult alpaca with a corneal perforation successfully treated with a conjunctival pedicle graft.

Lavage systems are used to facilitate the frequent administration of topical ophthalmic in animals that may be difficult to treat due to pain or behavior. Nasolacrimal lavage systems allow medications to be injected through 22-g polyethylene tubing traversing the nasolacrimal system from the nasal punctum to the lacrimal sac.[8] Commercially available subpalpebral lavage (SPL) systems, commonly used in horses, also may be used in camelids. Because of the concern for inducing iatrogenic corneal ulceration from the SPL footplate due to the camelid's tight-fitting eyelids, a modified SPL with a smaller footplate has been used. The SPL was well tolerated, the only complication noted was mild conjunctival irritation in one animal.[37]

Corneal disease in New World camelids is most often traumatic. To the author's knowledge, immune-mediated keratitis has not been reported in these animals and topical steroid administration should be used judiciously. Topical steroid administration may induce abortion, thus should be avoided in pregnant animals.[8]

SUMMARY

Diseases of the camelid ocular surface are common, and often due to trauma. Topical antimicrobials used for cases of conjunctivitis, keratoconjunctivitis, and ulcerative keratitis should be broad-spectrum. Cytology and cultures are performed as necessary.

REFERENCES

1. Kadwell M, Fernandez M, Stanley HF, et al. Genetic analysis reveals the wild ancestors of the llama and the alpaca. Proc Biol Sci 2001;268(1485):2575–84. ISSN 0962-8452. Available at: https://www.ncbi.nlm.nih.gov/pubmed/11749713.
2. Alpaca Owner's Association, I. Alpacas registered worldwide. Available at: https://www.alpacainfo.com/about/statistics/alpacas-worldwide.
3. Registry, I. L. Worldwide statistics: owners. Disponível em: Available at: https://secure.lamaregistry.com/registry-services/lama-statistics-owners.php.
4. Gionfriddo JR, Gionfriddo JP, Krohne SG. Ocular diseases of llamas: 194 cases (1980-1993). J Am Vet Med Assoc 1997;210(12):1784–7. ISSN 0003-1488. Available at: https://www.ncbi.nlm.nih.gov/pubmed/9187731.
5. Gelatt KN, Otzen Martinic GB, Flaneig JL, et al. Results of ophthalmic examinations of 29 alpacas. J Am Vet Med Assoc 1995;206(8):1204–7. ISSN 0003-1488. Available at: https://www.ncbi.nlm.nih.gov/pubmed/7768745.
6. Webb AA, Cullen CL, Lamont LA. Brainstem auditory evoked responses and ophthalmic findings in llamas and alpacas in Eastern Canada. Can Vet J 2006; 47(1):74–7. ISSN 0008-5286. Available at: https://www.ncbi.nlm.nih.gov/pubmed/16536233.
7. Gionfriddo JR. Update on llama medicine. Ophthalmology. Vet Clin North Am Food Anim Pract 1994;10(2):371–82. ISSN 0749-0720. Available at: https://www.ncbi.nlm.nih.gov/pubmed/7953968.
8. Gelatt KN, Gilger BC, Kern TJ, et al. Veterinary ophthalmology. Two-volume set. Chicester (England): Wiley; 2013. p. 2186, 1 online resource.
9. Fahmy MF, Arnautović I, Abdalla O. The morphology of the tarsal glands and the glands of the third eyelid in the one-humped camel. Acta Anat (Basel)

1971;78(1):40–6. ISSN 0001-5180. Available at: https://www.ncbi.nlm.nih.gov/pubmed/5555200.

10. Trbolova A, Gionfriddo JR, Ghaffari MS. Results of Schirmer tear test in clinically normal llamas (*Lama glama*). Vet Ophthalmol 2012;15(6):383–5. ISSN 1463-5224. Available at: https://www.ncbi.nlm.nih.gov/pubmed/22429698.

11. Mcdonald JE, Knollinger AM, Dees DD, et al. Determination of Schirmer tear test-1 values in clinically normal alpacas (*Vicugña pacos*) in North America. Vet Ophthalmol 2018;21(1):101–3. ISSN 1463-5224. Available at: https://www.ncbi.nlm.nih.gov/pubmed/28295997.

12. Gionfriddo JR, Melgarejo T, Morrison EA, et al. Comparison of tear proteins of llamas and cattle. Am J Vet Res 2000;61(10):1289–93. ISSN 0002-9645. Available at: https://www.ncbi.nlm.nih.gov/pubmed/11039563.

13. Gionfriddo JR, Davidson H, Asem EK, et al. Detection of lysozyme in llama, sheep, and cattle tears. Am J Vet Res 2000;61(10):1294–7. ISSN 0002-9645. Available at: https://www.ncbi.nlm.nih.gov/pubmed/11039564.

14. Shamsi FA, Chen Z, Liang J, et al. Analysis and comparison of proteomic profiles of tear fluid from human, cow, sheep, and camel eyes. Invest Ophthalmol Vis Sci 2011;52(12):9156–65. ISSN 1552-5783. Available at: https://www.ncbi.nlm.nih.gov/pubmed/22025569.

15. Wang Z, Chen Z, Yang Q, et al. Vitelline membrane outer layer 1 homolog interacts with lysozyme C and promotes the stabilization of tear film. Invest Ophthalmol Vis Sci 2014;55(10):6722–7. ISSN 1552-5783. Available at: https://www.ncbi.nlm.nih.gov/pubmed/25257056.

16. Chen Z, Shamsi FA, Li K, et al. Comparison of camel tear proteins between summer and winter. Mol Vis 2011;17:323–31. ISSN 1090-0535. Available at: https://www.ncbi.nlm.nih.gov/pubmed/21293736.

17. Sapienza JS, Isaza R, Johnson RD, et al. Anatomic and radiographic study of the lacrimal apparatus of llamas. Am J Vet Res 1992;53(6):1007–9. ISSN 0002-9645. Available at: https://www.ncbi.nlm.nih.gov/pubmed/1626768.

18. Gionfriddo JR, Rosenbusch R, Kinyon JM, et al. Bacterial and mycoplasmal flora of the healthy camelid conjunctival sac. Am J Vet Res 1991;52(7):1061–4. ISSN 0002-9645. Available at: https://www.ncbi.nlm.nih.gov/pubmed/1892259.

19. Storms G, Meersschaert C, Farnir F, et al. Normal bacterial conjunctival flora in the Huacaya alpaca (*Vicugna pacos*). Vet Ophthalmol 2016;19(1):22–8. ISSN 1463-5224. Available at: https://www.ncbi.nlm.nih.gov/pubmed/25581469.

20. Gionfriddo JR, Gabal MA, Betts DM. Fungal flora of the healthy camelid conjunctival sac. Am J Vet Res 1992;53(5):643–5. ISSN 0002-9645. Available at: https://www.ncbi.nlm.nih.gov/pubmed/1524286.

21. Tejedor-Junco MT, Gutiérrez C, González M, et al. Outbreaks of keratoconjunctivitis in a camel herd caused by a specific biovar of *Moraxella canis*. J Clin Microbiol 2010;48(2):596–8. ISSN 1098-660X. Available at: https://www.ncbi.nlm.nih.gov/pubmed/20032257.

22. Andrew SE, Ramsey DT, Hauptman JG, et al. Density of corneal endothelial cells and corneal thickness in eyes of euthanatized horses. Am J Vet Res 2001;62(4):479–82. ISSN 0002-9645. Available at: http://www.ncbi.nlm.nih.gov/pubmed/11327451.

23. Rankin AJ, Hosking KG, Roush JK. Corneal sensitivity in healthy, immature, and adult alpacas. Vet Ophthalmol 2012;15(1):31–5. ISSN 1463-5224. Available at: https://www.ncbi.nlm.nih.gov/pubmed/22051098.

24. Schuh 1991 CVJ.

25. Sandmeyer LS, Bauer BS, Breaux CB, et al. Congenital nasolacrimal atresia in 4 alpacas. Can Vet J 2011;52(3):313–7. ISSN 0008-5286. Available at: https://www.ncbi.nlm.nih.gov/pubmed/21629429.

26. Mangan BG, Gionfriddo JR, Powell CC. Bilateral nasolacrimal duct atresia in a cria. Vet Ophthalmol 2008;11(1):49–54. ISSN 1463-5216. Available at: https://www.ncbi.nlm.nih.gov/pubmed/18190353.

27. Brightman AH, Mclaughlin SA, Brumley V. Keratoconjunctivitis in a llama. Vet Med Small Anim Clin 1981;76(12):1776–7. ISSN 0042-4889. Available at: https://www.ncbi.nlm.nih.gov/pubmed/6915682.

28. Fischer K, Hendrix D. Conjunctivitis and ulcerative keratitis secondary to conjunctival plant foreign bodies in a herd of alpacas (*Lama pacos*). Vet Ophthalmol 2012;15(2):110–4. ISSN 1463-5224. Available at: https://www.ncbi.nlm.nih.gov/pubmed/22050866.

29. Gelatt KN. Congenital and acquired ophthalmic diseases in the foal. Anim Eye Res 1993;1(2):15–27.

30. Jones ML, Gilmour MA, Streeter RN. Use of grid keratotomy for the treatment of indolent corneal ulcer in a llama. Can Vet J 2007;48(4):416–9. ISSN 0008-5286. Available at: https://www.ncbi.nlm.nih.gov/pubmed/17494370.

31. Ledbetter EC, Montgomery KW, Landry MP, et al. Characterization of fungal keratitis in alpacas: 11 cases (2003-2012). J Am Vet Med Assoc 2013;243(11): 1616–22. ISSN 1943-569X. Available at: https://www.ncbi.nlm.nih.gov/pubmed/24261813.

32. Coster ME, Ramos-Vara JA, Vemulapalli R, et al. *Coccidioides posadasii* keratouveitis in a llama (*Lama glama*). Vet Ophthalmol 2010;13(1):53–7. ISSN 1463-5224. Available at: https://www.ncbi.nlm.nih.gov/pubmed/20149177.

33. Pirie CG, Pizzirani S, Parry NM. Corneal epithelial inclusion cyst in a llama. Vet Ophthalmol 2008;11(2):111–3. ISSN 1463-5224. Available at: https://www.ncbi.nlm.nih.gov/pubmed/18302575.

34. Pucket JD, Boileau MJ, Sula MJ. Calcific band keratopathy in an alpaca. Vet Ophthalmol 2014;17(4):286–9. ISSN 1463-5224. Available at: https://www.ncbi.nlm.nih.gov/pubmed/23998709.

35. Richter M, Grest P, Spiess B. Bilateral lipid keratopathy and atherosclerosis in an alpaca (*Lama pacos*) due to hypercholesterolemia. J Vet Intern Med 2006;20(6): 1503–7. ISSN 0891-6640. Available at: https://www.ncbi.nlm.nih.gov/pubmed/17186874.

36. Kiliç N, Toplu N, Aydoğan A, et al. Corneal papilloma associated with papillomavirus in a one-humped camel (*Camelus dromedarius*). Vet Ophthalmol 2010; 13(Suppl):100–2. ISSN 1463-5224. Available at: https://www.ncbi.nlm.nih.gov/pubmed/20840097.

37. Borkowski R, Moore PA, Mumford S, et al. Adaptations of subpalpebral lavage systems used for llamas (*Lama glama*) and a harbor seal (*Phoca vitulina*). J Zoo Wildl Med 2007;38(3):453–9. ISSN 1042-7260. Available at: https://www.ncbi.nlm.nih.gov/pubmed/17939355.

Ocular Surface Biology and Disease in Fish

David L. Williams, MA, MEd, VetMD, PhD, DECAWBM, CertVOphthal, CertWEL, FHEA, FRCVS

KEYWORDS

- Fish • Eye • Cornea • Biology • Disease

KEY POINTS

- Ensuring the clarity of the ocular surface of fish species with which we interact is of great importance.
- There is still much more to learn about the ocular surface of fish species.
- A better understanding of the anatomy, physiology, and pathology of the ocular surface is thus vital for fish welfare, as well as being a fascinating subject in its own right.

INTRODUCTION

The ocular surface of fish is different from that of terrestrial vertebrates in at least 3 major ways. First, although the ocular surface of an animal living in a land environment has to deal with the potential detrimental effects of drying and of physical and immunologic disturbances the fish eye, living in an aquatic environment has far fewer of these insults and so a somewhat different ocular surface anatomy and physiology from terrestrial animals. This means that the fish does not have to produce tears to lubricate its ocular surface. Having said that, the major insult faced by the ocular surface in fish is an osmotic one. For saltwater fish in the sea there is little of an osmotic challenge because the water in which they swim is relatively iso-osmolar with their cornea and the aqueous humor inside the anterior chamber. For freshwater fish, there is a continual osmotic gradient from the aqueous humor inside the eye to the water outside. How does the cornea deal with this continual potential water flux? Think then of the salmon, which in a few hours swims from the sea to its freshwater breeding grounds: how does the cornea cope with this challenge? Second, the cornea of all terrestrial animals provides a key refractive surface because light is passing from air to cornea and thence aqueous humor. In aquatic animals such as fish, the cornea plays no discernible role in refraction, meaning that it does not need to have as regular a corneal surface as eyes seeing in air. Streamlining of the ocular surface gives a

The author has nothing to disclose.
Department of Veterinary Medicine, University of Cambridge, Madingley Road, Cambridge CB3 0ES, UK
E-mail address: dlw33@cam.ac.uk

substantial astigmatism that has no refractive effect for the fish seeing underwater but may make fundoscopy somewhat difficult. Incidentally, this lack of corneal refractive power also means that the lens in fish is almost always spherical, because it provides the refractive element of the eye on its own. Third, although most terrestrial mammals grow to a defined adult size and then stop growing, with their eyes similarly reaching a specific adult size and then stopping developing further, fish often continue growing throughout life with their eyes also enlarging continually as the fish ages. This means that the cornea also increases in width and thickness throughout the fish's life. As we discuss the biology and diseases of the piscine ocular surface, we need to keep these peculiarities of the fish eye in mind. One might think that relatively little would be known of the fish ocular surface compared with that of more conventionally kept mammals. In fact, the zebrafish (*Danio danio*) has become a widely used model organism for all manner of diseases in humans and so its eye is remarkably well understood for such an apparently inconsequential animal, and at a morphologic and molecular level we are beginning to understand more of the teleost eye through work on *Danio*. A final point to note before we begin is that although we may like to think of fish as one discrete group of animals, from an evolutionary stance they are actually widely varying. We have teleosts, the conventional bony fish from goldfish kept as freshwater ornamental animals to the sea-dwelling cod, which we might eat, or the salmon, which migrates from freshwater to the sea and back again, but also the cartilaginous fish such as sharks and rays that evolved quite separately.

AN INTRODUCTORY REVIEW OF FISH EVOLUTION

Before we begin evaluating the piscine ocular surface, we must take a quick tour through the evolution of the group. Indeed, "fish" are a paraphyletic group not a distinct class of animals. The traditional classification and the modern classification are shown in **Table 1**. The term "fish" is normally used to describe a group of poikilothermic (cold-blooded) aquatic vertebrates in the Chordata phylum that breathe with gills. Scientifically we use the term "fish" to refer to Agnatha (jawless fishes), Chondrichthyes (sharks and rays), Sarcopterygii (lobe-finned fishes), and Actinopterygii (ray-finned fishes), but phylogenetically these classes of fish diverged evolutionarily at very different times; fish do not represent a monophyletic group. This is important when considering differences in anatomy of the ocular surface, as different fish have markedly varying corneal morphology and adnexal anatomy. The key groups we discuss are the primitive jawless fishes exemplified by the lamprey (*Lampetra planeri*), the cartilaginous Chondrichthyes, such as the sharks exemplified by the dogfish *Scliorhinus* and the bony Osteichthyes such as the teleosts, which are so widely varied it would be wrong to single out one species. There are benthic fish living on the sea floor, pelagic fish living in the midlevel water column, and fish living in the neritic or shallow-water zone. Each group has different ocular adaptations to their habitat across ocular anatomy but nowhere more important than in the ocular surface.

ANATOMY AND BIOLOGY OF THE FISH OCULAR SURFACE

The very fact that the ocular surface of the fish has to contend with a very different environment to that of the terrestrial mammal should alert us to the likelihood that its biology in health and disease may be significantly different from that we are used to in more conventional species encountered on a daily basis in our clinics.

Table 1 Classification of fish	
Traditional Classification	**Modern Classification**

• Class *Agnatha* (jawless fish)
  ○ Subclass *Cyclostomata* (hagfish and lampreys)
  ○ Subclass *Ostracodermi* (armored jawless fish)
• Class *Chondrichthyes* (cartilaginous fish)
  ○ Subclass *Elasmobranchii* (sharks and rays)
  ○ Subclass *Holocephali* (chimaeras and extinct relatives)
• Class *Placodermi* (armored fish)
• Class *Acanthodii* ("spiny sharks," sometimes classified under bony fishes)
• Class *Osteichthyes* (bony fish)
  ○ Subclass *Actinopterygii* (ray-finned fishes)
  ○ Subclass *Sarcopterygii* (fleshy-finned fishes, ancestors of tetrapods)
	• Class Myxini (hagfish)
	• Class *Pteraspidomorphi* (early jawless fish)
	• Class *Thelodonti*
	• Class *Anaspida*
	• Class *Petromyzontida* or *Hyperoartia*
	  ○ Petromyzontidae (lampreys)
	• Class *Conodonta* (conodonts)
	• Class *Cephalaspidomorphi* (early jawless fish)
	• Infraphylum *Gnathostomata* (jawed vertebrates)
	  ○ Class *Placodermi* (armored fish)
	  ○ Class *Chondrichthyes* (cartilaginous fish)
	  ○ Class *Acanthodii* (spiny sharks)
	  ○ Superclass *Osteichthyes* (bony fish)
	    ■ Class *Actinopterygii* (ray-finned fish)
	      • Subclass *Chondrostei*
	        ○ Order *Acipenseriformes* (sturgeons and paddlefishes)
	        ○ Order *Polypteriformes* (reedfishes and bichirs).
	      • Subclass *Neopterygii*
	        ○ Infraclass *Holostei* (gars and bowfins)
	        ○ Infraclass *Teleostei* (many orders of common fish)
	    ■ Class *Sarcopterygii* (lobe-finned fish)
	      • Subclass *Actinistia* (coelacanths)
	      • Subclass Dipnoi (lungfish)

EYELIDS AND CONJUNCTIVA

Sharks have well-developed eyelids, although these move little and do not cover the surface of the eye entirely apart from in nurse sharks (*Ginglymostoma* species) and swell sharks (*Cephaloscyllium* species), both of these being bottom-dwelling fish that hunt through the seabed, hence requiring a protective eye-closure reflex.[1] Other sharks, such as the requiem sharks (Carcharhinidae) and hammerheads (Sphyrnidae), have nictitating membranes that can themselves completely cover the cornea when required. Where it is present, a complex series of 5 muscles act together to draw the nictitating membrane backward and upward over the globe, the principal one of which is the levator palpebrae nictitans, which is also involved with opening the spiracle. Teleost eyes are in many cases partly covered with thickened tissue folds or adipose lids formed as lateral ingrowth from the circumocular sulcus. Sometimes these skin folds join to form a spectacle covering the eye entirely and necessarily being fully transparent. The lids of the Mullet *Mugil* are particularly bulbous through the lipid they contain, whereas in the mackerel *Scomber* this accretion of lipid occurs only during the breeding season. The herring has lids with a fibrous plexus organized so that it is birefringent and may act to allow the fish to recognize polarized light.[2] Lids that form a complete spectacle over the globe may act to filter out harmful ultraviolet wavelengths of light in shallow-dwelling fish, as we shall see later in birefringent cornea. The lids of many fish species often contain mucus-secreting cells that take us to a consideration of tear production in fish. Clearly animals dwelling underwater have no need for aqueous tears and as such do not have lacrimal glands. Nevertheless, they have goblet cells in the conjunctiva of their lids and in the cornea in some cases that produce considerable amounts of mucus, which, as we will see later may have significant beneficial effects in the eye already immersed in water.

CORNEA

As with all vertebrates, the fish cornea is composed of an epithelium, a stroma, a Descemet membrane, and an endothelium. There are several differences between the fish cornea and that of the mammal, and even between different species of fish. The first is that in many, but not all species of fish the epithelium makes up approximately half of the thickness of the cornea. This may be to prevent movement of water between the stroma and the external environment or possibly as a mechanism to limit the effects of corneal trauma in fish where eyelids do not protect the eye, although there does not appear to be a correlation between epithelial thickness and presence or absence of eyelids. Second, different fish species have different types of spectacle. Walls[3] considers there to be 3 types of spectacle. The first, seen in lampreys, is a transparent covering of lid skin across the ocular surface, quite separate from the underlying cornea. The spectacle in such fish has an external epithelium of 4 to 7 layers contiguous with the skin epithelium. The secondary spectacle of Walls[3] forms when the dermal cornea is separated from the underlying scleral cornea with a subspectacular space traversed by a layer of connective tissue, as in the eel and other benthic species, which, being bottom-dwellers, require protection of the corneas in much the same way as snakes burrowing underground in the early part of their evolution benefited from their spectacles. Walls'[3] tertiary spectacles form in pelagic species in which the eyelids fuse to create a covering with a true subspectacular space lined with conjunctival epithelium as particularly reported in anchovies (*Engraulis*), milkfish (*Chanos*),[4] and threadfins (*Polydactylus*).

The lamprey has a stroma of approximately 40 lamellae, with vertically orientated fibers between lamellae binding them together and then a posterior epithelium of its own which, although it has a thin electron-dense layer, has no Descemet membrane. The cornea proper, as it were, lies underneath with its own epithelium, stroma, and endothelium (**Fig. 1**). The epithelium here though is a single layer

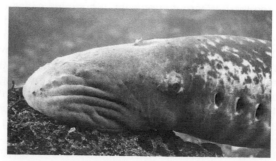

Fig. 1. The spawning lamprey and its edematous cornea.

of cells with a well-developed rough endoplasmic reticulum. The epithelial surface is generally composed of hexagonal cells but with round to oval cells interspersed between them with numerous microplicae. The most marked feature, though, is the presence of numerous large micro-holes of approximately 400 nm in diameter, through which mucous granules are expelled onto the corneal surface. The stroma has several lamellae arranged orthogonally to one another external to a true Descemet membrane as the basement membrane of the endothelium. The 2 structures are separated by a mucoid layer. During spawning, the lamprey spectacle becomes opaque, rendering the fish blind for a period (**Fig. 2**). Although this change in the snake is merely occasioned by water influx as the newly generated spectacle separates from the old structure, in the lamprey, there is an influx of leukocytes that break down the anterior stroma. Indeed, research has shown that blindness does not affect the migration of lampreys during their breeding season,[5] as it appears that detection of pheromones is more important in this behavior.

The elasmobranchs, exemplified by the sharks, have a cornea and indeed a globe as a whole, that is oval-shaped with a long axis streamlined and more highly curved than that of most other fish genera. As we noted in the introduction, this astigmatism would be a significant problem in a terrestrial animal but in one existing in an aquatic environment the difference in curvature of the cornea in the horizontal and vertical axis makes no difference with regard to refraction where the cornea does not act as a refractive surface. The epithelium comprises approximately half of the corneal thickness. The surface cells of the stratified squamous epithelium have numerous microplicae (**Fig. 3**). The double stroma, superficially a dermal element and deeper a scleral component (**Fig. 4**) has numerous collagen fibrils embedded in a gelatinous proteoglycan matrix much as the mammalian cornea but one major difference is the presence of sutural fibers binding the stromal lamellae together, either as fine fibrils binding the entire stroma together from the Bowman layer superficially to the Descemet membrane at depth, diagonal fibers spanning 2 or 3 lamellae only or as thicker fibers crossing only a few lamellae at a time. These sutural fibers are key in preventing stromal swelling in these fish that do not possess an endothelial layer actively pumping water out of the stroma into the anterior chamber.[6] To put some numerical data on the bare bones of this histologic variation, the swelling pressure in the spiny dogfish

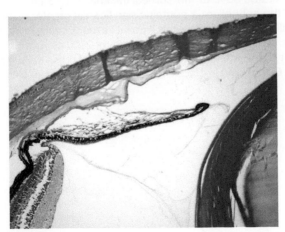

Fig. 2. Histology of the cornea and anterior segment of the lamprey. ($\times$ 80 haematoxylin and eosin).

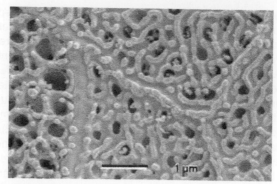

Fig. 3. Scanning electron microscopy of the surface of black shark cornea showing microplicae.

Squalus acanthias is less than 10 mm Hg in normal levels of hydration compared with a figure of 60 mm Hg in the rabbit cornea.[7] The reason for this difference in response to immersion in water may lie in the much thicker epithelium in these sharks (**Fig. 5**) and many other fish, which stops water entering the stroma. The relevance of this in the living marine shark may be to explain how these animals, in a similar fashion to the migrating lamprey discussed earlier, can swim considerable distances up freshwater rivers in search of food without their corneal transparency being affected by the considerable difference in osmotic gradient between fresh and salt water and the corneal stroma.

THE TELEOST CORNEA

We noted previously that we would use the research undertaken on the zebrafish (*Danio* sp) to exemplify the fish cornea, but this is only possible for teleosts of which *Danio* is a member. The thickness of the zebrafish cornea is only 20 μm, compared with that of the dog or cat at between 350 and 450 μm, but it contains what appears at first sight to be the normal layers we are used to in the dog or cat: epithelium, stroma, and endothelium. Truth be told, that is rather a simplification: the teleost cornea differs from the canine cornea in several respects. First the epithelium of the zebra *Danio* constitutes 60% of the corneal thickness (12.5 μm). This is common to most fish, where the epithelium a contains significantly greater number of cell layers than any mammalian corneal epithelium.[8] Epithelial cell density is highly varied across species: the trout, for instance, has a cell density of 2300 cells/mm², whereas the sea robin has a density of 40,800 cells/mm². The surface of these cells is characterized by microridges (**Fig. 6**) that hold in place mucus produced by goblet cells, the openings of

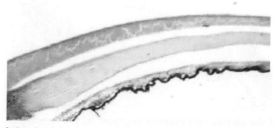

Fig. 4. Histology of the double cornea of a shark. (×120 haematoxylin and eosin).

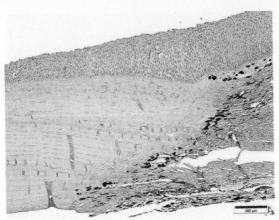

Fig. 5. Histology showing the thick corneal epithelium of a shark. (haematoxylin and eosin).

which can be seen on the ocular surface (**Fig. 7**). This mucus covering protects the cornea from damage, but if this occurs it can be visualized with fluorescein dye just as in the dog or cat (**Fig. 8**).

Second, the teleost stroma is composed of 2 distinct stromas, a dermal element and a scleral element, separated by a mucoid layer. Anterior stroma forms what is known in human ophthalmology as the Bowman layer, an acellular zone of stroma, also seen in other higher apes and in some avian species. Edelhauser and Siegesmuns[9] suggest that this stromal layer may serve as an additional barrier to the osmotic difference between the freshwater environment and the aqueous humor, although there seems little correlation between the presence or absence of the Bowman layer and the environment in which the particular species lives. Many teleostean corneas have colored filters, giving a yellow hue to the cornea as they absorb light at the more damaging blue end of the spectrum. Some fish have occlusable corneas in which these filters change depending on light illumination levels.[10] It appearance that the melanophores change their light-transmitting capability by changing pigment migration associated with microtubules in chromatophores. Other corneal stromas exhibit birefringence, whereby a significant proportion of the light is reflected, this is particularly seen in fish inhabiting shallow waters where ultraviolet radiation is intense, as we discuss further later in this

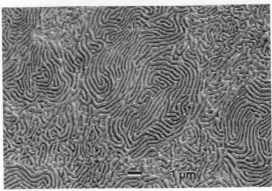

Fig. 6. Scanning electron microscopy of the ocular surface of a dover sole showing microridges.

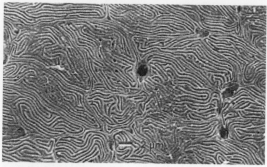

Fig. 7. Scanning electron microscopy of a bar-tailed flathead showing the openings of mucus-secreting goblet cells.

article.[11] The birefringence occurs though changes in the refractive index of sequential layers of the stromal collagen lamellae.[12] Collin has suggested a number of different structures giving rise to birefringence from connective tissue in the cornea stroma, amorphous material between corneal lamellae, stacks of collagen fibrils within the stroma, aligned rough endoplasmic reticulum within keratocytes or layers of whole cells aligned in the stroma, each of these occurring in different species; clearly such an effect reflecting light back away from the eye has evolved a number of times and must be of value in a range of different fish.[13]

As with any biological system, there will be cases that exist on their own as remarkable exceptions to normal anatomy. With regard to the fish cornea, it is the sandlance that stands apart from any other species. As a burrowing fish that hunts small prey species locating them by moving its eyes independently while keeping its body still under the substrate, its cornea has a phenomenally expanded stroma, giving the cornea a high refractive power even with a relatively flat lens. As noted earlier, the refractive power of most piscine corneas is exceptionally limited and the lens, relatively large and spherical, performs most of the ocular refraction. The same is not true of the sandlance, in which the refractive index of the refractive lenticule in the posterior corneal stroma is 1.38 compared with the refractive index of a marine fish such as the flounder of 1.36 and surrounding seawater at 1.34. Such a small

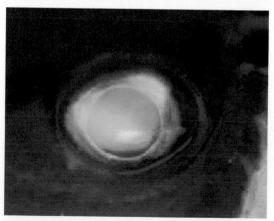

Fig. 8. The cornea of a fish with a corneal abrasion stained with fluorescein

difference may not seem particularly relevant, but the size and shape of the stromal lenticule gives up to 200 diopters of focusing power. A lens-shaped area in the center of the stroma of the pipefish, *Coryrthoichthys paxtoni,* filled with a granular material of similar high refractive index, may provide a similar refractive function, but this has yet to be proven.[14]

PHYSICAL TRAUMA AND HEALING OF THE FISH OCULAR SURFACE

The corneas of some benthic fish, and in particular sturgeon and stingrays, are often seen to be to varying degrees opaque through abrasive lesions. These species are particularly prone to such posttraumatic disease as they do not have spectacles. In pearlfish of the *Carapus* genus, the cornea becomes progressively more damaged with age and becomes opaque except in species such as *Carapus* and *Encheliophis* species that protect themselves by being parasitic in the anus of sea cucumbers.[15]

One of the problems of detecting physical trauma and resulting epithelial damage in aquatic animals is that the differences in the ocular surface between terrestrial mammals and fish may lead to variation in the effects of such compounds as fluorescein, regularly used to detect epithelial erosions in mammals and local anesthetics such as tetracaine. One article investigating the use of unbuffered tricaine and fluorescein in Nile tilapia (*Oreochromis niloticus*) and channel catfish (*Ictalurus punctatus*) showed that the pH of the topical mixture can cause changes in epithelial uptake of the dye even if not frank epithelial erosion, thus potentially leading to erroneous diagnosis of corneal ulceration where damage is not at full epithelial thickness.[16]

ULTRAVIOLET LIGHT DAMAGE OF THE FISH OCULAR SURFACE

Any eye is whatever species experience somewhat on a conundrum with regard to damage by rays of the electromagnetic spectrum. The very reason for existence of the eye is to see light, and yet photons themselves can damage tissues to the point of rendering them opaque. The lens has various mechanisms of reducing such damage, through the antioxidant effects of glutathione[17] to the chaperone effects of alpha crystallin, the major structural protein of the lens.[18] The cornea has different ways of reducing the effects of ultraviolet radiation, and indeed one of its prime functions is to filter out such short wavelength radiation to limit lenticular and retinal oxidative damage. One might expect that ultraviolet-related damage would be less in an aquatic organism such as a fish than in a terrestrial mammal because water attenuates the passage of UV radiation. Yet fish swimming in shallow water in areas with high levels of sunlight can experience levels of UV irradiation relatively similar to a terrestrial animal in the same latitude. Coral reef fish are particularly prone to such sunburn, if we can use a colloquial term for this UV-related damage, with one report showing that fish on the Great Barrier Reef experience up to 30 times the minimal erythemal dose capable of causing sunburn in people.[19] Marine organisms may use behavioral strategies to limit such damage, living under rocks or in caves, but also synthesize or sequester compounds in or on the ocular surface that act as sunscreens by absorbing UV rays.[20] The problem with absorbing such photons within the tissues of the ocular surface is that the absorbed energy then needs to be dispersed and this causes opacifying damage to the necessarily regular protein filaments of the cornea. Better would be a mechanism that absorbed this damaging irradiation in the tear film itself, which is continually produced and lost from the ocular surface. UV-absorbing mycosporinelike amino acids within mucins of the piscine ocular surface provide exactly the absorptive photospectrum required.[21] The only problem is that these amino acids cannot be produced by vertebrates and thus need to be gained by trophic transfer from marine invertebrates. Tropical marine fish use 4 such amino acids, palythine, palythene, palythinol, and austerina-300, together with gadusol, a UVB-absorbing compound.[22] Interestingly, the nutritive absorption of such compounds from prey is not merely passive. At least in the reef fish the Hawaiian saddleback wrasse, *Thalassoma duperrey*, the UV absorption of ocular surface mucus increases when the fish are exposed to UV irradiation, but only when a dietary source of these sunscreen compounds is available.[23] The mechanism by which such changes in mucus composition occurs is unclear. The lens blocks UV radiation from reaching the retina so a photoreceptor-related mechanism is unlikely. It may be that pineal-related UV absorption changes the release of these UV-absorbing compounds from storage depots given the rapid changes seen in mucus composition when fish are exposed to UV radiation.

OCULAR SURFACE PATHOLOGY IN GAS SUPERSATURATION

Fish kept in situations of gas supersaturation through inappropriate water pumping mechanisms can develop exophthalmia and intraocular or intrastromal gas bubbles with associated ocular surface pathology.[24] The same can occur in fish normally living at depth where a countercurrent mechanism in the blood vessels of the choroid generates high partial pressures of oxygen. When farmed in shallow water the gas can come out of solution as gas bubbles as we have shown in farmed halibut[25,26] and Smiley and colleagues have demonstrated in sea bass.[27]

MICROBIAL PATHOGENS ON THE FISH OCULAR SURFACE

We know relatively little of viral diseases of the fish ocular surface. The ranavirus causing mortality in largemouth and smallmouth bass populations is one however where ocular disease is well recognized. Exophthalmos together with dermal and corneal erosions and ulcers are seen in moribund fish in which histopathologically a widespread panuveitis occurs with associated keratitis (**Fig. 9**). There is a heterophilic necrosis predominantly involving the ciliary body and choroid but the inflammatory cells may dissect under Descemet membrane causing perforating ulcers, severe conjunctivitis and episcleritis.[28] Disease of milkfish (*Chanos chanos*) in the Philippines was attributed to *Vibrio harveyi*[29] and corneal opacification developing in the common

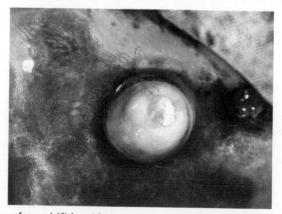

Fig. 9. The cornea of a goldfish with panophthalmitis showing the degree of ulcerative keratitis.

snook (*Centropomus undecimalis*) shortly after capture[30] was associated with *V harveyi*. Without treatment, the fish became blind. Similarly, eye lesions in the short sunfish (*Mola mola*), which were attributed to aggression by other fish, were colonized by *V harveyi*.[31]

PARASITIC DISEASE OF THE OCULAR SURFACE

Parasitic disease in the fish eye is well recognized with trematode metacercariae noted in the lens of a number of fish species, blinding the animals and thus changing their behavior to reside nearer the water surface allowing birds to catch and eat them, fulfilling the parasite life cycle.[32] Damage to the eye does not seem to form part of the lifecycle of the copepods parasitizing the ocular surface of the sharks in which they may cause partial or complete blindness. Having said that, we know significantly less about the parasitic copepod *Ommatokoita elongata,* which affects Pacific sleeper sharks with potentially devastating visual effects, than we do about the cataractogenic trematodes mentioned previously. In both deep sea Pacific sleeper sharks, *Somniosus pacificus,* and in Greenland sharks, *Somniosus microcephalus,* only female copepods or copepod larvae have been found embedded in the corneal epithelium of both eyes, whereas similar infestations of *Phrixocephalus cincinnatus* in the arrowhead flounder, *Atheresthes stomias,* are normally affected only unilaterally and then mostly in the right eye.[33] This parasitic tendency may be related to the method of infection, and the lack of bilaterally affected fish may be linked to a high mortality in this species while sleeper sharks, relying less on their vision, are affected to a lesser extent by visual dysfunction. Perhaps the unilaterality of infestation in the flounder noted earlier relates to the migration of the eye in this flatfish, clearly an area for further research!

The microsporidian *Tetramicra brevifilum* causes morbidity and mortality in a number of host species, such as turbot, with parasitic cysts giving exophthalmos as part of widespread pathology. In the lumpfish, an important cleaner fish species used in aquaculture as biological control for copepod parasites in salmon species, *Tetramicra* causes exophthalmos and white blisters on the ocular surface filled with flocculent material shown cytologic and with electron microscopy to consist of microsporidial sporoblasts.[34] The disease described in the lumpfish was severe with widespread xenomas around and within the eye as well as elsewhere in the body. While Matthews and Matthews suggested that affected turbot could recover,[35] welfare considerations might suggest that euthanasia was more appropriate.

These 2 examples of parasitic disease affecting the ocular surface are by no means meant to be given as the only instances in which parasites affect the cornea, but merely to demonstrate that where researchers have taken the tie to document the changes seen in the ocular surface where parasites affect the eye, plenty can be learned. All that remains is for future researchers to investigate more thoroughly other instances of parasitism damaging the ocular surface.

TOXIC EFFECTS ON THE OCULAR SURFACE

Fish are particularly vulnerable to the effects of toxic pollutants and it is perhaps surprising that more reports are not extant in the literature regarding toxic effects of compounds on the ocular surface. The report by Uppal and colleagues[36] on toxic effects of the organophosphate herbicide monocrotophos on the ocular surface of the zebrafish *Cyprinus carpio communis* thus serves as a good example of the use of this species as a model for ocular surface toxicity of other compounds in varying species. Toxicity here, even at sublethal doses involved shrinkage of the microridges on the epithelial surface and the formation of crystalloid structures within the epithelial cells with subsequent necrosis. As has been widely recognized for many years, the corneal epithelium rapidly reconstitutes itself after most physical trauma with ready capability of wound healing and ocular surface renewal.[37] Yet, when after 30 days of exposure to monocrotophos the fish were transferred to a noncontaminated environment, the epithelium failed to return to its normal morphology even after a further 60 days.

GENETIC DEFECTS OF THE FISH OCULAR SURFACE

I include this paragraph not because we have a large amount of information on genetic defects in the fish ocular surface, but rather for the opposite reason. With the zebrafish genome now sequenced and the opportunity for site-directed mutagenesis being used by several laboratories, evaluation of inherited corneal defects is likely to grow exponentially in the next few years.

OCULAR SURFACE BIOLOGY OF *ANABLEPS*, HALF IN HALF OUT OF THE WATER!

Given the difference in corneas of fish inhabiting varying environments, one would expect perhaps that *Anableps*, the "4-eyed" fish that lives at the very water surface with half its eye above water and half below (**Fig. 10**) would have 2 ocular surfaces quite different in morphology. The refractive power of the combined ocular surface and lens are significantly different for the portions of the eye above and below water; the cornea above water is thin, as is seen in terrestrial vertebrates, whereas that below the water surface is thicker, as seen in totally aquatic fish. On the other hand, research from Collin's group has shown a substantial similarity between the 2 ocular surfaces themselves (**Fig. 11**).[38] In terms of cell density (16,387 ± 3995 cells per mm^2 above water compared with 22,428 ± 6387 cells per mm^2 below water) and micro-ridge morphology, the 2 corneas did not vary significantly. The key to this is in observing the animal's behavior. The fish *Anableps microlepis* have been noted to dip their heads under the water 2 to 4 times each minute.[39] In this way, the fish manages to keep its ocular surface lubricated as if it were underwater. Even so, one might expect that a fish that has existed for long enough to evolve a globe with such marked refractive differences above and below the water level might have also evolved an ocular surface adapted to life in air rather than water. The evidence, apart from corneal thickness, which relates to its refractive power, suggests not.

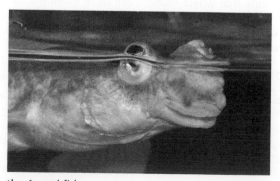

Fig. 10. *Anableps*, the 4 eyed fish.

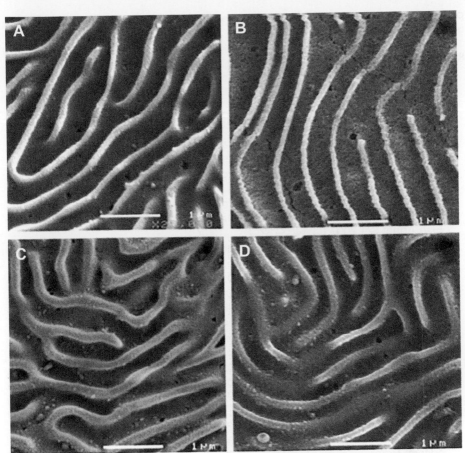

Fig. 11. The similarity of corneal epithelial surfaces above (*A*, *B*) and below (*C*, *D*) water.

SUMMARY

It might have been recognized by the reader that at the end of most of the preceding paragraphs, we have noted that there are still questions to be answered and research to be undertaken to answer the questions posed in this review. Certainly, we know a decent amount regarding the ocular surface of many fish species, and work by groups, such as those run by Barry and Shaun Collins and Russell Fernald, has extended this substantially. Yet a short review such as this one merely serves, in its author's opinion at least, to show how much more there is still to learn about the ocular surface of such a vast range of species, living in such varied environments, as do fish species globally. Vision is so important in most fish species that ensuring the clarity of the ocular surface of fish species with which we interact is of great importance. A better understanding of the anatomy, physiology, and pathology of the ocular surface is thus vital for fish welfare, as well as being a fascinating subject in its own right.

ACKNOWLEDGMENTS

The author wishes to thank many zoologists and ichthyologists for their assistance with his interest in the piscine eye over the years and especially Dr Collin for permission to use Figures 3, 6, 7 and 11 and Professor R Dubielzig for permission to use Figures 2, 4 and 5.

REFERENCES

1. Nicol JA, Somiya H. The eyes of fishes. Oxford (United Kingdom): Oxford University Press; 1989.
2. Stewart KW. Observations on the morphology and optical properties of the adipose eyelid of fishes. J Fish Res Board Can 1962;19(6):1161–2.
3. Walls GL. The vertebrate eye and its adaptive radiation. Bloomsbury Hills (MI): The Cranbrook Institute of Science; 1942.
4. Chang CH, Chiao CC, Yan HY. The structure and possible functions of the milkfish *Chanos chanos* adipose eyelid. J Fish Biol 2009;75:87–99.
5. Binder TR, McDonald DG. Is there a role for vision in the behaviour of sea lampreys (*Petromyzon marinus*) during their upstream spawning migration? Can J Fish Aquat Sci 2007;64:1403–12.
6. Keller N, Pouliquen Y. Ultrastructural study of the posterior cornea of the dogfish "*Scyliorhinus canicula L*". Cornea 1985;4:108–17.
7. Edelhauser HF, Hoffert JR, Fromm PO. A comparative study of sodium permeability in lake trout and rabbit corneas. Am J Physiol 1968;214:389–94.
8. Zhao XC, Yee RW, Norcom E, et al. The zebrafish cornea: structure and development. Invest Ophthalmol Vis Sci 2006;47:4341–8.
9. Edelhauser HF, Siegesmund KA. The localization of sodium in the teleost cornea. Invest Ophthalmol 1968;7(2):147–55.
10. Siebeck UE, Collin SP, Ghoddusi M, et al. Occlusable corneas in toadfishes: light transmission, movement and ultrastruture of pigment during light- and dark-adaptation. J Exp Biol 2003;206(13):2177–90.
11. Collin HB, Collin SP. The cornea of the sand lance, *Limnichthyes fasciatus* (Creeiidae). Cornea 1988;7(3):190–203.
12. Land MF. The physics and biology of animal reflectors. In: Butler JAV, Noble D, editors. Progress in biophysics and molecular biology, vol. 24. Oxford (England): Pergamon Press; 2014. p. 77–106.
13. Collirt SP, Collin HB. The fish cornea: adaptations for different aquatic environments. Sensory biology of jawed fishes: new insights. 2001. p. 57–96.
14. Collin HB, Collin SP. Ultrastructure and organisation of the cornea, lens and iris in the pipefish, *Corythoichthyes paxtoni* (Syngnathidae, Teleostei). Histol Histopathol 1995;10(2):313–24.
15. Parmentier E, Vandewalle P. Morphological adaptations of pearlfish (Carapidae) to their various habitats. Fish adaptations. 2003. p. 261–76.
16. Davis MW, Stephenson J, Noga EJ. The effect of tricaine on use of the fluorescein test for detecting skin and corneal ulcers in fish. J Aquat Anim Health 2008;20(2):86–95.
17. Giblin FJ. Glutathione: a vital lens antioxidant. J Ocul Pharmacol Ther 2000;16:121–35.
18. Horwitz J. Alpha-crystallin. Exp Eye Res 2003;76:145–53.
19. Shick JM, Dunlap WC. Mycosporine-like amino acids and related gadusols: biosynthesis, accumulation, and UV-protective functions in aquatic organisms. Annu Rev Physiol 2002;64(1):223–62.
20. Jokiel PL. Solar ultraviolet radiation and coral reef epifauna. Science 1980;207(4435):1069–71.
21. Cockell CS, Knowland J. Ultraviolet radiation screening compounds. Biol Rev Camb Philos Soo 1000;74:311–15.

22. Zamzow JP. Effects of diet, ultraviolet exposure, and gender on the ultraviolet absorbance of fish mucus and ocular structures. Mar Biol 2004;144:1057–64.
23. Banaszak AT, Lesser MP. Effects of solar ultraviolet radiation on coral reef organisms. Photochem Photobiol Sci 2009;8:1276–94.
24. Hoffert J, Fromm P. Biomicroscopic, gross and microscopic observations of the corneal lesions in the lake trout *Salvenlinus namaycuch*. J Fish Res Board Can 1965;22:761–6.
25. Williams DL, Wall AE, Branson E, et al. Preliminary findings of ophthalmological abnormalities in farmed halibut. Vet Rec 1995;136:610–2.
26. Williams DL, Brancker W. Intraocular oxygen tensions in normal and diseased eyes of farmed halibut. Vet J 2004;167(1):81–6.
27. Smiley JE, Okihoro MS, Drawbridge MA, et al. Pathology of ocular lesions associated with gas supersaturation in white seabass. J Aquat Anim Health 2012;24: 1–10.
28. Boonthai T, Loch TP, Yamashita CJ, et al. Laboratory investigation into the role of largemouth bass virus (*Ranavirus*, Iridoviridae) in smallmouth bass mortality events in Pennsylvania rivers. BMC Vet Res 2018;14(1):62.
29. Ishimaru K, Muroga K. Taxonomical re-evaluation of two pathogenic *Vibrio* species isolated from milkfish and swimming crab. Fish Pathol 1997;32:59–64.
30. Kraxberger-Beatty T, McGarey DJ, Grier HJ, et al. *Vibrio harveyi*, an opportunistic pathogen of common snook, *Centropomus undecimalis* (Bloch), held in captivity. J Fish Dis 1990;13(6):557–60.
31. Austin B, Zhang XH. *Vibrio harveyi*: a significant pathogen of marine vertebrates and invertebrates. Lett Appl Microbiol 2006;43(2):119–24.
32. Ashton N, Brown N, Easty D. Trematode cataract in fresh water fish. J Small Anim Pract 1969;10:471–8.
33. Kabata Z. *Phrixocephalus cincinannatus* (Wilson 1908 *Copepoda* Lemaeoceridae): morphology, metamorphosis and host-parasite relationship. J Fish Res Board Can 1969;26:921–34.
34. Scholz F, Fringuelli E, Bolton-Warberg M, et al. First record of *Tetramicra brevifilum* in lumpfish (*Cyclopterus lumpus, L.*). J Fish Dis 2017;40:757–71.
35. Matthews RA, Matthews BF. Cell and tissue reactions of turbot *Scophthalmus maximus (L.)* to *Tetramicra brevifilum* gen. n., sp. n. (Microspora). J Fish Dis 1980;3:495–515.
36. Uppal RK, Johal MS, Sharma ML. Toxicological effects and recovery of the corneal epithelium in *Cyprinus carpio communis Linn.* exposed to monocrotophos: an scanning electron microscope study. Vet Ophthalmol 2015;18:214–20.
37. Buck RC. Cell migration in repair of mouse corneal epithelium. Invest Ophthalmol Vis Sci 1979;18:767–84.
38. Simmich J, Temple SE, Collin SP. A fish eye out of water: epithelial surface projections on aerial and aquatic corneas of the 'four-eyed fish' *Anableps anableps*. Clin Exp Optom 2012;95(2):140–5.
39. Schwassmann HO, Kruger L. Experimental analysis of the visual system of the four-eyed fish *Anableps microlepis*. Vision Res 1965;5:269–81.

Ocular Surface Biology and Disease in Amphibians

David L. Williams, MA, MEd, VetMD, PhD, DECAWBM, CertVOphthal, CertWEL, FRCVS

KEYWORDS

- Ocular surface • Amphibians • Vision • Eye • Corneal lipidosis

KEY POINTS

- Vision is essential for amphibians, so a healthy ocular surface is critically important.
- There are ocular surface abnormalities that occur predominantly in captive animals, such as corneal lipidosis, whereas there are others, such as UV-induced trauma or infectious and parasitic conditions, that may be critical to survival for animals in the wild.
- It is believed that inherited defects are going to be seen in small captive populations but it may be that confined wild groups of amphibians can be just as severely affected.
- Anything that blinds an animal severely affects its life changes, showing how important the ocular surface is to the welfare of individual amphibians and the conservation of populations as a whole.

INTRODUCTION

At the end of my paper in this volume 'Ocular surface biology and disease in fish' it was noted that Anableps the 'four eyed fish' differs in its corneal thickness for the part of its cornea above the water surface versus that below. Apart from that, however, its ocular surfaces are surprisingly similar given the very different local environments with which they interact. That fish Is able to maintain this similarity by keeping its dorsal cornea moist at all times. The amphibian inhabits both terrestrial and aquatic environments but its eye, however, needs to change at different stages in its life from that of the wholly aquatic tadpole to the eye of the adult frog or salamander which needs to cope with the demands of the above-water environment. It has been noted in the discussion of the ocular surface of fish[1] that the epithelium of the cornea in wholly aquatic species was generally far thicker than that of terrestrial animals, with the squamous epithelium of fifteen or more layers compared to perhaps five in corneas exposed to the air. Are similar differences seen between the corneal epithelia of aquatic amphibians and more terrestrial species? And

The author has nothing to disclose.
Department of Veterinary Medicine, University of Cambridge, Madingley Road, Cambridge CB3 0ES, UK
E-mail address: dlw33@cam.ac.uk

Vet Clin Exot Anim 22 (2019) 97–107
https://doi.org/10.1016/j.cvex.2018.08.008
1094-9194/19/© 2018 Elsevier Inc. All rights reserved.

what changes are seen between the universally aquatic larval stages and adults after metamorphosis?

Do amphibians have ocular surface diseases specifically related to the differences in environment encountered in different life stages? And what diseases affect the cornea in its larval and adult stages? This article aims to answer these questions, but I fear coming up with more new questions than answers. It is nearly 25 years since I wrote, with Dr Brent Whittaker, a review of the amphibian eye,[2] and, truth to tell, we have sadly made few advances in understanding the amphibian ocular surface since then. Perhaps this article can be a wake-up call for working harder to study this structure, especially in light of threats to amphibian health and welfare from UV light exposure with environmental change to the potential catastrophe of chytrid fungal infection.[3]

ANATOMY AND PHYSIOLOGY OF THE LARVAL AND ADULT AMPHIBIAN

There are few research articles on the morphology of the amphibian ocular surface given that most interest has lain in details of the retina and neural architecture of the amphibian eye rather than its more anterior structures.[4] Those articles on the cornea of amphibians have focused on it physiology and many have focused on using the frog cornea as a model for studying ion transfer.[5,6] They are thus not particularly relevant to clinical questions of amphibian ophthalmic structure, function, and disease although even in some older reports useful descriptions of corneal structure are provided.[7]

Ironically one of the most complete reports of the ocular surface in a specific amphibian species is that of the *Xenopus* eye, but this species is aquatic in both its larval and adult forms (**Figs. 1–3**). That being the case, *Xenopus* does not have fully formed upper and lower eyelids or lacrimal glands although, along with other amphibians, does have a harderian gland. The optic vesicle develops at stage 25 (giving ages of developing amphibia is inappropriate because, their being poikilotherms, their speed of development varies with temperature), and at this point the cornea is formed of 2 layers, 1 a superficial embryonic epidermis with goblet cells and ciliated cells and the other a basal embryonic epidermal layer that receives signals from the developing retina underneath, which encourage it to develop into a lens. This transdifferentiation remains an option throughout life and removal of the lens stimulates corneal cells to develop into a new lens. Embryonic lens differentiation starts at stage 30 and is finished by stage 35, at which point the lens detaches and the anterior chambers forms. At stages 37 to 39, the corneal endothelium forms but at stage 41 a new stream of cells migrates in the forming stroma. A clear space forms between the superficial cornea and the deep layer rather mirroring the double-layered corneas seen in some fish species. It seems that the inner cornea is formed from neural crest cells whereas the outer cornea is predominantly ectodermal in origin. At stages 48 to 50, active stromal cell migration occurs toward the so-called stromal attracting center (**Fig. 4**). Stage 62 signals metamorphosis in *Xenopus* and in the same way that the cells of the tail undergo apoptosis as it disappears, so the cells of the stromal attracting center apoptose, leaving a thin stroma overlain by a 10-cell to 13-cell thick epidermis. By 2 years of age, full adulthood, the stroma is approximately 70-μm to 80-μm thick, approximately 65% of corneal thickness. As discussed previously, *Xenopus* does not have fully formed eyelids but does have a lower membrane that forms over the eye and its opening signals major changes in the ocular surface[8] with maturation of epithelium and stroma and an increased proliferation rate of the relevant cell populations.

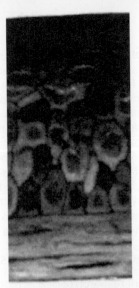

Fig. 1. Histology of the *Xenopus* tadpole with the majority of the cornea comprised of epithelium.

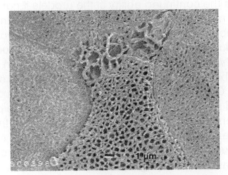

Fig. 2. Scanning electron microscopy of the ocular surface of an axolotl showing wide variation in cell surface morphology.

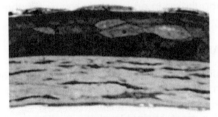

Fig. 3. Histology of the adult *Xenopus* frog with a much thinner epithelium.

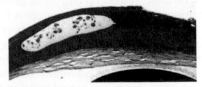

Fig. 4. Histology of the cells of the stromal attracting center undergoing apoptosis during metamorphosis.

What then of terrestrial amphibians? Ultrastructural changes in the cornea of *Rana pipiens*, the leopard frog, are significantly more marked—eyelids form together with the nictitating membrane and Harderian glands. The numbers of ciliated cells on the cornea and developing lids increase but in the adult frog cilia are lost but the epithelium is perforated by numerous openings of cutaneous glands and goblet cells.[9] Histology of the tree frog *Hyla orientalis* cornea shows a much thinner epidermis in the adult animal[10] A study on another anuran with prominent eyes, *Pleurodema*, shows a cornea comprising an epithelium of 3-5 cells thick but comprising a full one-third of the corneal thickness with the stroma the other two-thirds, so considerably more than a mammalian epithelium.[11] The larval stage G40, however, aquatic as it is, has an epithelium that is more than half of the corneal thickness. At stage G41, the upper and lower eyelids and the nictitating membrane begin to form to provide protection for the cornea and allow the epithelium to provide a less a defensive guard.

EMBRYOLOGIC DEFECTS OF THE AMPHIBIAN OCULAR SURFACE

There is little in the way of recent research or clinical reports of embryologic ocular defects in amphibians. That was not the case a century ago when Warren Harmon Lewis produced a series of articles on the development of the anuran eye,[12–14] although his particular interest was the continued ability of the urodele if not the anuran cornea to dedifferentiate into a new lens. Lewis would have been fascinated by what is now known of the remarkable conservation of activity of the pax6 homeobox gene across huge swathes of evolutionary time, with mutations affecting ocular development in species from *Drosophila* to mammals and humans.[15,16] Given this similarity across species, it should not be a surprise that *Xenopus* pax6 mutants show microphthalmia, aniridia, and cataract. Given that pax6 is also key in generation of the limbal stem cell population,[17] it should not be a surprise from an ocular surface perspective that such mutants also have corneal clouding from keratopathy. Does this have relevance to wild populations? One fascinating example of what might be caused by inbreeding comes from the introduced Cururu toads (*Rhinella jimi*) on the archipelago of Fernando de Noronha off the coast of Brazil (**Fig. 5**).[18,19] These animals have a variety of malformations from microcephaly and anophthalmia to bragnathia and brachydactyly. More specifically, regarding the ocular surface, many affected animals have palpebral deformities, keratitis, and corneal opacities. Whether these are merely the effect of inbreeding in a small population in an isolated area or whether UV light or pesticides also have a part to play is unclear.

TRAUMA AND CORNEAL WOUND HEALING IN AMPHIBIANS

Experimental work on corneal wound healing has been reported using the amphibian cornea as a model from the very early studies on epithelial migration in ulcer healing[20] through to recent studies on matrix metalloproteinase enzyme involvement in corneal wound restoration.[21] At a more clinical level, the problems with corneal ulceration in amphibians are complicated by the difficulty in protecting the ocular surface with topical lubricants as might be used in a dog or cat,[22] inappropriate to use in an animal living in a highly humid environment, or tarsorrhaphy, or a third eyelid flap, which is regularly used to protect the ocular surface by veterinarians in companion animal species although not necessarily recommended by veterinary ophthalmologists.[23] Thus healing of corneal ulceration in amphibians can be a lengthy process and, as with so much of exotic animal practice, the key is prevention before treatment, and optimal husbandry is key in ensuring adequate humidity and avoiding environmental stressors (**Fig. 6**).

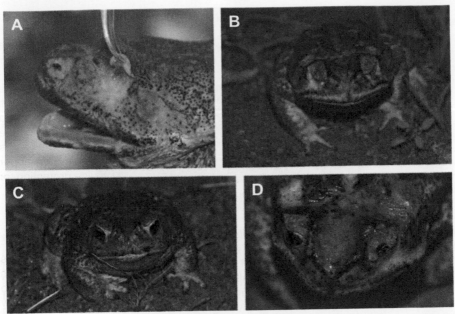

Fig. 5. Ocular abnormalities in *Rhinella jimi*. (*A*) Anophthalmos in the left eye; (*B*) Eyelids fused to skin with bilateral anophthalmos; (*C*) Corneal opacity in left eye; (*D*) Deformed eyelids. (*Courtesy of* Drs LP and RS Toledo.)

The exposure of the amphibian ocular surface given the paucity of eyelid coverage of the cornea in many anuran species might suggests that UV light could cause epithelial damage to the amphibian ocular surface.[24] Phototoxic keratitis as seen in people is characterized by ocular pain, tearing, conjunctival chemosis, blepharospasm, and deterioration of vision typically occurring several hours after exposure in mountaineers, skiers, or arc weld workers.[25] The problem in amphibians is a much more chronic one of lower-dose UV exposure but has been seen more in captive animals kept in environments with added UV lighting (**Fig. 7**). A study by Novales Flamarique and

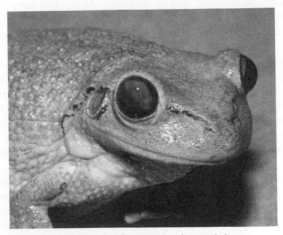

Fig. 6. Corneal ulcer in a frog shown by fluorescein dye staining.

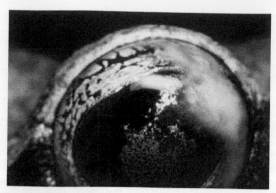

Fig. 7. UV irradiation–associated corneal scarring in a tree frog.

colleagues[24] examined tadpoles of *Hyla regilla*, the Pacific chorus frog, and *Rana aurora*, the northern red-legged frog, in a forest clearing near Victoria in British Columbia, Canada, reared in 3 different regimes: ambient sunlight, sunlight blocked for wavelengths under 450 nm, and sunlight enhanced at 280 nm to 320 nm. Several *R aurora* individuals reared in these enhanced conditions developed lens opacities but also skin and corneal opacities. The investigators note that the removal of riparian vegetation and increase in UV-B exposure of small water bodies where amphibians would spawn may give a higher prevalence of UV-related injuries. They suggest that "monitoring the incidents of cataracts [and ocular surface lesions – DLW] in clear-cuts and forest pools could potentially be used as an indicator of biological effects of increased UV-B radiation."[24(p187)]

INFECTIOUS AND PARASITIC DISEASE

Bacterial panophthalmitis, including conjunctivitis, has been reported in leopard frogs *Rana pipiens* infected with *Flavobacterium* indologenes[26] and in fire-bellied toads with a mixed gram-negative infection.[27] Helman and colleagues[28] reported parasitic conjunctivitis and lacrimal adenitis in *Ambystoma tigrinum mavortium*, tiger salamanders, caused by a spirurid nematode, which resulted in periocular fluctuate swellings eventually preventing eyelid opening. At postmortem examination, the epithelial lining of the lacrimal gland ducts and conjunctiva were hyperplastic and the ducts contained multiple nematode larvae with morphologic features character-istic of a spirurid. A further report of ocular surface lesions, such as ulcerative kera-titis in rhabditid nematode–associated ophthalmitis and meningoencephalomyelitis in captive Asian horned frogs (*Megophrys montana*),[29] shows that the eye may be a focus of disease in any parasite with visceral larva migrans as a mechanism in its pathogenesis. These case reports are likely only to be the tip of the iceberg of infec-tious and parasitic disease affecting the ocular surface—the fact that these case re-ports have been published should not lead to considering that these are sole instances but merely individual examples of much wider disease in wild, if not captive, animals.

Other reports have documented keratitis in wild amphibian populations not associ-ated with any pathogens but seen in conjunction with dehydration, lethargy, and hind limb paralysis. The animals were found as part of a survey for *Batrachochytrium den-drobatidis*, a chytrid fungus causing the panzootic disease chytridiomycosis, but goes to show what other disease entities might be discovered were scientists to examine wild populations in more detail. The animals in this instance were either dead or moribund and thus euthanized on welfare grounds.[30]

LIPID KERATOPATHY IN AMPHIBIANS

Perhaps the most remarkable ocular surface condition in captive amphibians is that of corneal lipidosis. First reported in 1986 by Carpenter and colleagues,[31] the xanthomatous keratitis, as the investigators termed it, was part of a more generalized lipid deposition in an adult female Cuban tree frog (*Osteopilus sepentrionalis*), at the Museum of Science in Boston, fed day-old mice but was a sole lipid lesion in 2 Cuban tree frogs in Lincoln Park Zoo in Chicago fed crickets and mealworms. Postmortem analysis of the amphibian from Boston showed extracellular cholesterolosis staining with oil red O with a granulomatous reaction extending into the ciliary body. The brain was replaced by a xanthoma originating in the third ventricle and one in the hypothalamus. The liver was devoid of pathologic xanthomatosis but did contain abundant lipid. Atherosclerosis was noted in the aorta and femoral arteries and skeletal muscles were affected by motor atrophy and small xanthomas associated with nerves. The 2 frogs from Lincoln Park Zoo had similar corneal lesions to the Boston animal but no extraocular xanthomas or atherosclerosis. Serum lipid analysis showed cholesterol at 196 mg/dL and 201 mg/dL, triglycerides at 84 mg/dL and 94 mg/dL, high-density lipoproteins at 22 mg/dL and 25 mg/dL, and low-density lipotproteins at 62 mg/dL and 65 mg/dL for the 2 Lincoln Park frogs. Russell and colleagues[32] reported similar findings in 5 female Cuban tree frogs of 8 held in Tulsa Zoological Park in Oklahoma. These animals became blind, lost weight, and were either euthanized or died. No treatments were found to be successful. Cholesterol levels were 683 mg/dL and 791 mg/dL and triglyceride levels were 86 mg/dL and 47 mg/dL. Two surviving frogs developed milder signs of corneal lipidosis with slight bilateral involvement in a male frog and a more severe unilateral involvement in a female frog. Necropsies showed generalized xanthomatosis. Other breeds including the Cuban knight anole[31] and I have seen the condition in several White's tree frogs. Millichamp and colleagues[33] also reported the condition in White's tree frogs. Shilton and colleagues[34] fed Cuban tree frogs a high-cholesterol diet with this lipid making up 1.5% of the diet's dry matter. They observed signs of corneal lipidosis or xanthomatosis in only 9 months on this diet with both arcus lipoides corneae and concomitant hypercholesterolemia in about half of the frogs. None of the control frogs was similarly affected. This study demonstrated a significant elevation in circulating lipids, including very low-density lipoprotein, low-density lipoprotein, and high-density lipoprotein cholesterol, in these experimental frogs. But what is the cause of the condition in captive frogs not experimentally fed a high fat diet? To begin, it was believed that perhaps these animals were indeed being fed a high fat diet—the Boston proband was fed day-old mice, with stomachs full of milk. Perhaps this was the reason for the lipidosis? Yet other animals have been fed crickets and meal worms; diet cannot be the only factor. It was believed, given the female preponderance of affected frogs, that these individuals may be mobilizing cholesterol before spawning. Perhaps if an appropriate spawning site is not available, this higher circulating lipid might deposit itself in the cornea. Yet the fact that male frogs can be affected mean that this cannot be the full answer. The life history of a captive anuran is very different from that of the same species in the wild. Wild male anurans spend much time and energy in calling with an estimate made that a 5-g frog consumes approximately 1.5 mL O_2/g/h.[34] Captive animals simply do not have this need to expend energy. There is a big difference between an animal in captivity and one in the wild and, as with everything in exotic animal medicine, having

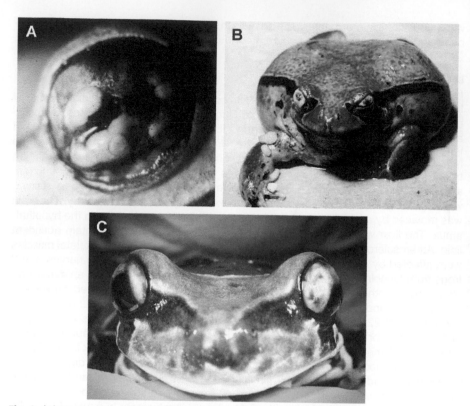

Fig. 8. (*A*) Lipid keratopathy in a White's tree frog. (*B*) Lipid keratopathy in a tomato frog. (*C*) Lipid keratopathy in a mission golden-eyed tree frog. (*Courtesy of* Dr Brey Moore.)

captivity mirror the wild as closely as possible is the key to successful life health and welfare of the animals. And perhaps that is a good place to end this survey of the ocular surface of amphibians showing how well linked the anatomy, physiology, and pathology of the ocular surface are to the welfare of individual amphibians and conservation of populations as a whole (**Figs. 8 and 9**).[35]

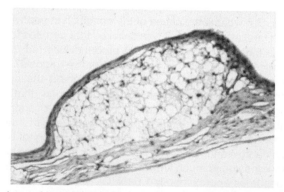

Fig. 9. Histopathology of lipid keratopathy showing lipid infiltrate in stroma immediately under the epithelium.

SUMMARY

Vision is essential for amphibians, so a healthy ocular surface is critically important. There are ocular surface abnormalities that occur predominantly in captive animals, such as corneal lipidosis, whereas there are others, such as UV-induced trauma or infectious and parasitic conditions, that may be critical to survival for animals in the wild. It is generally believed that inherited defects are likely to be seen in small captive populations but it may be that confined wild groups of amphibians can be just as severely affected. Anything that blinds an animal severely affects its life changes, showing how important the ocular surface is in the welfare of individual amphibians and the conservation of populations as a whole.

ACKNOWLEDGMENTS

A review article such as this is never just the work of the authors but brings together what I have learnt through many others over the years. I gratefully acknowledge Professor John E Cooper, Drs Steve Barten and Fred Frye and to Dr Luis Felipe Toledo for permission to use the images in Figure 5 and Dr Wanzhou Hu for permission to use the images in Figures 1, 3 and 4.

REFERENCES

1. Kafarnik C, Fritsche J, Reese S. In vivo confocal microscopy in the normal corneas of cats, dogs and birds. Vet Ophthalmol 2007;10:222–30.
2. Williams DL, Whitaker BR. The amphibian eye: a clinical review. J Zoo Wildl Med 1994;18–28.
3. Pasmans F, Canessa S, Martel A. The eye of the storm: silent infections driving amphibian declines. Anim Conserv 2018;21:102–3.
4. Hoskins SG. Metamorphosis of the amphibian eye. J Neurobiol 1990;21(7): 970–89.
5. Zadunaisky JA. Active transport of chloride in frog cornea. Am J Physiol 1966; 211:506–12.
6. Chalfie M, Neufeld AH, Zadunaisky JA. Action of epinephrine and other cyclic AMP-mediated agents on the chloride transport of the frog cornea. Invest Ophthalmol Vis Sci 1972;11:644–50.
7. Kaye GI. Studies on the cornea: III. The fine structure of the frog cornea and the uptake and transport of colloidal particles by the cornea in vivo. J Cell Biol 1962; 15(2):241–58.
8. Wiechmann AF, Wirsig-Wiechmann CE, Wirsig-Wiechmann CR. Color atlas of Xenopus laevis histology. New York: Springer Science & Business Media; 2003.
9. Kaltenbach JC, Harding CV, Susan S. Surface ultrastructure of the cornea and adjacent epidermis during metamorphosis of Rana pipiens A scanning electron microscopic study. J Morphol 1980;166(3):323–35.
10. Akat E, Arikan H. A histological study of the eye in Hyla orientalis (Bedriaga, 1890) (Anura, Hylidae). Biharean Biol 2013;7(2):61–3.
11. Volonteri C, Barrasso DA, Cotichelli L, et al. Eye ontogeny in P leurodema bufoninum: a comparison with P leurodema somuncurense (Anura, Leptodactylidae). J Morphol 2017;278(7):896–906.
12. Lewis WH. Experimental studies on the development of the eye in amphibia. I. On the origin of the lens. Rana Palustris. Am J Anat 1904;3:505–36.
13. Lewis WH. Experimental studies on the development of the eye in amphibia. II. On the cornea. J Exp Zool 1905;2:431–46.

14. Harmon Lewis W. Experimental studies on the development of the eye in amphibia. III. On the origin and differentiation of the lens. Am J Anat 1906;6: 473–509.

15. Gehring WJ. The master control gene for morphogenesis and evolution of the eye. Genes Cells 1996;1:11–5.

16. Hanson I, Van Heyningen V. Pax6: more than meets the eye. Trends Genet 1995; 11:268–72.

17. Collinson JM, Chanas SA, Hill RE, et al. Corneal development, limbal stem cell function, and corneal epithelial cell migration in the Pax6+/− mouse. Invest Ophthalmol Vis Sci 2004;45:1101–8.

18. Toledo LF, Ribeiro RS. The archipelago of Fernando de Noronha: an intriguing malformed toad hotspot in South America. EcoHealth 2009;6:351–7.

19. Tolledo J, Toledo LF. Blind toads in paradise: the cascading effect of vision loss on a tropical archipelago. Journal of Zoology 2015;296:167–76.

20. Arey LB, Covode WM. The method of repair in epithelial wounds of the cornea. Anat Rec 1943;86(1):75–86.

21. Carinato ME, Walter BE, Henry JJ. Xenopus laevis gelatinase B (Xmmp-9): development, regeneration, and wound healing. Dev Dyn 2000;217(4):377–87.

22. Williams DL, Wirostko BM, Gum G, et al. Topical cross-linked HA-based hydrogel accelerates closure of corneal epithelial defects and repair of stromal ulceration in companion animals. Invest Ophthalmol Vis Sci 2017;58:4616–22.

23. Van Der Woerdt A. Adnexal surgery in dogs and cats. Vet Ophthalmol 2004;7: 284–90.

24. Novales Flamarique I, Ovaska K, Davis TM. UV-B induced damage to the skin and ocular system of amphibians. Biol Bull 2000;199:187–8.

25. Cullen AP. Photokeratitis and other phototoxic effects on the cornea and conjunctiva. Int J Toxicol 2002;21:455–64.

26. Olson ME, Gard S, Brown M, et al. Flavobacterium indologenes infection in leopard frogs. J Am Vet Med Assoc 1992;201:1766–70.

27. Brooks DE, Jacobson ER, Wolf ED, et al. Panophthalmitis and otitis interna in fire-bellied toads. J Am Vet Med Assoc 1983;183(11):1198–201.

28. Helman RG, Barrie MT, Gardiner CH. Parasitic conjunctivitis and lacrimal adenitis in two tiger salamanders, Ambystoma tigrinum mavortium. Bull Assoc Rept Amph Vet 1998;8(1):9–12.

29. Imai DM, Nadler SA, Brenner D, et al. Rhabditid nematode-associated ophthalmitis and meningoencephalomyelitis in captive Asian horned frogs (Megophrys montana). J Vet Diagn Invest 2009;21:568–73.

30. Sunje E, Pasmans F, Maksimovic Z, et al. Recorded mortality in the vulnerable Alpine salamander, Salamandra atra prenjensis (Amphibia: Caudata), is not associated with the presence of known amphibian pathogens. Salamandra 2018;54:75–9.

31. Carpenter JL, Bachrach A Jr, Albert DM, et al. Xanthomatous keratitis, disseminated xanthomatosis, and atherosclerosis in Cuban tree frogs. Vet Pathol 1986; 23:337–9.

32. Russell WC, Edwards DL Jr, Stair EL, et al. Corneal lipidosis, disseminated xanthomatosis, and hypercholesterolemia in Cuban tree frogs (Osteopilus septentrionalis). J Zoo Wildl Med 1990;1:99–104.

33. Millichamp NJ, Dziezyc J, Anderson RE, et al. Lipid keratopathy in frogs: histopathology and biochemistry. Invest Ophthalmol Vis Sci 1990;15:542.

34. Shilton CM, Smith DA, Crawshaw GJ, et al. Corneal lipid deposition in Cuban tree frogs (Osteopilus septentrionalis) and its relationship to serum lipids: an experimental study. Journal of Zoo and Wildlife Medicine 2001;32(3):305–19.
35. Wright K. Cholesterol, corneal lipidosis, and xanthomatosis in amphibians. Vet Clin North Am Exot Anim Pract 2003;6:155–67.

Ocular Surface Disease in Reptiles

Kathryn M. Smith Fleming, DVM, PhD, DACVO

KEYWORDS

- Reptile • Ocular surface • Cornea • Spectacle • Ocular disease

KEY POINTS

- Anatomic variation exists between the eyes of lizards, chelonians, snakes, and crocodilians.
- A thorough ocular examination, physical examination, and clinical history are invaluable to obtaining a diagnosis and implementing treatment.
- Most ocular disease in reptiles is related to improper husbandry or trauma—proper client education is the key to prevention.
- Reading literature on the same or a related species is beneficial in identifying ocular lesions and disease in your patient.
- The intact spectacle prevents topical medications from reaching the cornea and globe.

INTRODUCTION

Much knowledge has been gained in the last 75 years regarding the anatomy and physiology of the reptilian eye in states of health and disease. That being said, much interspecies variation exists, especially when comparing snakes with Chelonia. Having a basic understanding of health and disease is important in preparing to examine a reptile. Therefore, the goal of this article is to serve as a central database of information on pertinent anatomy and ocular surface diseases reported in the literature for the main orders of reptiles.

OCULAR EXAMINATION

As with any species, examination of the ocular surface in reptiles begins with observations made at a distance with the animal freely moving (if possible). Abnormalities detected, such as an eyelid lesion or corneal opacity, can help you plan your detailed examination and gather any diagnostic supplies needed before restraining the animal. In this manner, you make the examination more efficient and reduce patient

Disclosure Statement: The authors have nothing to disclose.
Department of Veterinary Clinical Medicine, University of Illinois at Urbana-Champaign, 1008 West Hazelwood Drive, Urbana, IL 61802, USA
E-mail address: kmf5@illinois.edu

Vet Clin Exot Anim 22 (2019) 109–121
https://doi.org/10.1016/j.cvex.2018.08.006
1094-9194/19/© 2018 Elsevier Inc. All rights reserved.

vetexotic.theclinics.com

stress. Your distance examination should include evaluation of adnexal and ocular surface structures as much as possible. You should also observe visual behaviors such as feeding and/or navigating a known enclosure as well as an unknown environment, if possible. Just like dogs and cats, reptiles can adapt to vision loss well by mentally mapping a known space, making it difficult to detect chronic visual defects. However, in a novel environment, such as at the veterinary clinic or in a holding area, behaviors may be strikingly different. Attention should be paid to the animal's pace and head position when navigating a space because a unilateral vision deficit may cause the animal to turn its head or body such that the good eye is toward any object or perceived threat worth investigating. Animals with vision deficits may move more slowly or cautiously, have difficulty locating live prey, or bump into objects on the affected side (look for evidence of trauma). Bilaterally reduced vision may be more likely to result in behavior changes, whereas unilateral vision deficits may be more difficult to detect.

In order to examine the ocular surface in detail, restraint should be performed such that the handler, patient, and veterinarian are kept safe, the patient's head is as still as possible, and stress to the patient is minimized. For recommendations on proper animal restraint, practitioners should consult appropriate reference material or involve in the examination an exotic animal practitioner experienced in working with these species.[1,2] Once restrained, ocular reflex testing can be carried out in routine fashion. Some reptiles lack eyelids, therefore menace response in these animals will result in withdrawal of the head and palpebral reflex will be absent. Subsequently, a detailed examination of the eye should be completed, beginning with the adnexa and ocular surface and ending with a fundic examination. As with any species, the reptile ocular surface should be examined first in a well-lit room with a focal light source (penlight, transilluminator, etc.), before the examination is repeated in a dark room to highlight subtle lesions. A source of magnification (loupes, slit lamp biomicroscope, direct ophthalmoscope) should be available for the examination because lesions can be subtle and reptile eyes are often small. Species with a large and mobile nictitating membrane, such as crocodilians, can be difficult to examine when the membrane is elevated.[3] Using a cotton-tipped applicator or muscle hook can be helpful to retract it.

Diagnostic testing of the ocular surface, including fluorescein staining and tear film evaluation, have been described and should be carried out when indicated and possible. Ophthalmic stains such as fluorescein stain and rose bengal are useful in species with exposed cornea but not helpful in those with a spectacle.[4] Patency of the lacrimal duct can be assessed via direct application of stain to the ocular surface in most reptiles or via careful injection of 0.05 mL of fluorescein stain via 30 g needle into the subspectacular space under magnification.[4,5] In either case, fluorescein stain should be observed exiting the roof of the mouth if the duct is patent. Chelonians lack a lacrimal duct, therefore tears and fluorescein stain naturally spill over onto the face.[4]

Ocular surface disease can occur on its own or in conjunction with intraocular disease; therefore, a thorough and complete ocular examination is important and should be carried out when possible. Ocular examination findings should also be interpreted in the context of a full physical examination, because ocular manifestations of systemic disease are not uncommon among reptiles.[4]

A thorough and detailed history can be extremely beneficial in identifying possible causes or exacerbating factors of ocular surface disease in reptiles. Owners should be asked questions regarding the animal source, housing conditions, diet and supplement composition and source, previous medical history, and whether or not other animals are kept in the same enclosure or environment as the patient. It can also be helpful to know whether or not other animals in the enclosure or room are similarly affected.

THE REPTILE EYE

Although the basic layout of the eye is conserved across species, variation in ocular appearance, anatomy, and physiology among reptile orders can be striking. This is likely related to variation in evolutionary origin and environmental pressures.[6] Reptiles are classified into 5 main orders, 4 of which are more commonly encountered in veterinary medicine: lizards, chelonians, crocodilians, and snakes. Within the orders, groups (suborders and families) were formed based on anatomic and evolutionary traits. In general, animals in the same suborder or family group will share many similarities. Therefore, if literature is not available on the exact species a practitioner is examining, exploring texts related to animals in the same group may be beneficial.[4]

The remainder of the article has been divided into sections for ease of reference and includes 4 orders of reptiles: lizards, chelonians, crocodilians, and snakes. Within these sections you may find information on ocular surface anatomy and disease.

LIZARDS
Anatomy

Detailed descriptions of the reptilian eye can be found in several excellent references.[6–8] For the purposes of this article, the focus of the discussion will be ocular surface.

Most lizards have 2 eyelids with the lower being more mobile than the relatively fixed upper eyelid. In some species, the lower eyelid is relatively transparent and in others contains a cartilaginous tarsal plate.[4,6,7] Conjunctiva lines the underside of the eyelids, forms fornices as in mammals, and lines the globe before terminating at the limbus. A nictitating membrane, consisting of a fold of conjunctiva containing 3 cartilaginous flaps, can be raised over the corneal surface through contraction of the bursalis muscle pulling on an associated tendon.[6]

As with snakes, a few groups of lizards are ablepharine, where the eyelids have fused, become transparent, and formed a spectacle that overlays the cornea. These animals include the spectacled and Pygopodidae geckos, the wall lizard genus *Ophisops*, several species of skinks (*Ablepharus* sp, *Typhlacontias* sp), and worm lizards.[6,8] Those animals with spectacles also lack a nictitating membrane.[7] See the snake section for more detailed information about spectacles. Chameleons lack a nictitating membrane and have a much reduced palpebral fissure.[6,7]

Lizards possess 2 lacrimal openings and canaliculi on the lower eyelid near the medial canthus. These join together to form the nasolacrimal duct that travels anteriorly to open on the roof of the mouth. Several structures contribute to the lizard tear film, including the large Harderian gland, a mucoserous gland associated with the nictitating membrane, and a posteriorly located lacrimal gland. In addition, mucous secretion occurs in several areas of the palpebral conjunctiva.[6] In species with a spectacle, the lacrimal gland is typically absent and Harderian gland secretions are released between the cornea and spectacle.[6]

The lizard cornea is relatively thin and contains a thin surface epithelium, thick Bowman's layer, and thin stroma, Descemet's membrane, and endothelium. Corneal size relative to overall globe size varies greatly between lizard species.[6]

Ocular Surface Diseases

Conjunctivitis

Bacterial conjunctivitis was reported in 3 lizards in a zoologic collection, having isolated *Morganella*, *Pseudomonas*, *Acinetobacter*, *Staphylococcus*, and *Serratia* spp.[9] All isolates were susceptible to gentamicin and enrofloxacin and variably susceptible to fusidic acid in vitro, but clinical response did not always follow in vitro results. An outbreak of *Aeromonas liquefaciens* occurred in a laboratory colony of lizards resulting in conjunctivitis and mucopurulent discharge that sealed the eyelids shut.[10] The infection source could not be identified and systemic and topical therapies were often unrewarding.

Reptiles, unlike mammals, have heterophils that lack lysosomes; therefore, mucopurulent ocular discharge is not a typical finding in bacterial conjunctivitis. Rather, conjunctival plaque formation can occur.[4,11] Thorough examination of the conjunctival fornices should be performed on any animal with blepharospasm and ocular discharge and any conjunctival plaques encountered removed for cytologic analysis.[4]

Hypovitaminosis A

Several lizard species are susceptible to hypovitaminosis A, including leopard geckos, chameleons, and green anoles.[12–14] Leopard geckos seem unable to convert β-carotene, a common ingredient in many reptile multivitamins, to vitamin A and deficiency can result when they are given the incorrect supplement.[12] Early signs include blepharospasm, decreased tear production, and mucoid ocular discharge. Over time, the eyelids become swollen shut and thick, keratinous debris accumulates on the ocular surface. Diagnosis is typically based on clinical signs and supportive history. Diet change can be implemented in early cases, typically reversing clinical signs. More severely affected cases can be anesthetized such that keratinous debris can be flushed away and topical antibiotic ointment applied. Parenteral vitamin A supplementation will typically correct ocular changes in 2 to 4 weeks unless the patient has already decompensated systemically.[12] Several green anoles developed thickened lips and eyelids, histologically revealed as squamous metaplasia, keratinization, and decreased goblet cell density in the conjunctiva, consistent with lesions associated with hypovitaminosis A.[13] Samples were clear of infectious agents. Chameleons given low levels of vitamin A developed similar signs as discussed earlier.[14]

Miscellaneous causes

Certain tropical plants (*Ficus*, *Pothos* spp) contain oxalates within and as a white residue on the leaves and are commonly used in chameleon enclosures. Conjunctivitis has been reported in animals exposed to oxalate residue.[14] Misting plant leaves several times daily will reduce oxalate buildup. Keeping chameleons in well-ventilated wire cages is also beneficial.

CHELONIANS

Anatomy

The palpebral fissure in all chelonians is tilted, with the lateral canthus higher than the medial, likely related to head position when at the water's surface.[6] Similar to lizards, the lower eyelid is mobile but instead lacks cartilage.[6,7] Chelonians also possess a nictitating membrane that is lowered by the pyramidalis muscle.[6]

The lacrimal gland is large in marine turtles and those found in brackish water and is known to secrete salt.[6,15,16] Chelonians also possess a Harderian gland but lack a lacrimal duct.

Chelonians have a thick corneal epithelium compared with other reptiles. They also lack Bowman's membrane but have a thin Descemet's membrane and a thick endothelium. The convexity of the cornea varies greatly among species, likely related to an amphibious or terrestrial lifestyle.[17,18]

Ocular Surface Diseases

Conjunctival foreign bodies

Terrestrial chelonians kept on substrates such as hay or sand frequently suffer from conjunctival foreign bodies. Animals with blepharospasm and excess ocular discharge should undergo a thorough conjunctival examination and flushing of the conjunctival fornices with eye wash or balanced salt solution through a fine gauge cannula or intravenous catheter.[4] Larger foreign bodies can be manually removed with forceps.

Conjunctivitis

Bacterial conjunctivitis was reported in 2 tortoises in a zoologic collection from which *Staphylococcus*, *Corynebacterium*, and *Branhamella* spp were isolated.[9] All isolates were susceptible to gentamicin and cefuroxime, with variable susceptibility to fusidic acid. Both tortoises improved on topical fusidic acid with or without systemic enrofloxacin therapy.[9] *Mycoplasma* spp. were reported to cause ocular discharge and conjunctivitis in combination with respiratory disease in the gopher tortoise and Eastern box turtle.[19,20]

Reptiles, unlike mammals, have heterophils that lack lysosomes; therefore, mucopurulent ocular discharge is not a typical finding in bacterial conjunctivitis. Rather, conjunctival plaque formation can occur.[4,11] Thorough examination of the conjunctival fornices should be performed on any animal with blepharospasm and ocular discharge and any conjunctival plaques encountered removed for cytologic analysis.[4]

Parasitic conjunctivitis is well reported in chelonians. Leeches (*Ozobranchus* sp) have been found in green sea turtles.[3] Several *Neopolystoma* spp have been isolated from the conjunctival sac of freshwater chelonians, but the overall parasite burden is typically low.[21,22] A herpes-like virus infection resulted in conjunctivitis, ocular discharge, necrotizing stomatitis, and death in a group of Argentine and red-footed tortoises.[23]

Lung-eye-trachea disease

Conjunctivitis with caseous plaque formation is a known component of herpes virus–related lung, eye, and trachea disease in green sea turtles.[3] Animals may also have caseous exudate covering the eyes. Secondary bacterial conjunctivitis with gram-negative bacteria often ensues, creating a keratoconjunctivitis.[24] The disease can also cause corneal opacification or plaque formation. Affected animals may make gasping sounds, which indicate respiratory involvement, and may be unable to dive. Clinical lesions can seem similar to those of early vitamin A deficiency.[11]

Fibropapilloma of sea turtles

Herpes virus infection of green sea turtles and loggerhead turtles can cause ocular lesions affecting the cornea, eyelids, periocular skin, and conjunctiva as well as other cutaneous and even visceral locations.[25] Lesions are proliferative, ulcerated masses that are sessile or on a stalk and possess a cauliflower-like surface of hyperplastic epithelium overlying areas of reactive fibroblasts. Secondary infection, usually gram-negative bacteria, can make matters worse. Surgical mass removal may be attempted but recurrence is common given the viral cause. Infected individuals can also spread virus to others. Lesion appearance is quite characteristic and supports the diagnosis but biopsy provides a definitive answer.[4]

Fibroma, fibropapilloma, and fibrosarcoma have been reported to develop on the eyelids and conjunctiva of green sea turtles due to a proliferative response to trematode eggs.[3,26] The parasite, *Laeredius laeredii*, releases eggs into the bloodstream, where they lodge in small vessels of the skin and conjunctiva.

Corneal lipid

Corneal arcus lipoides, a white band of cholesterol crystals in the peripheral, perilimbal cornea, can be seen in *Testudo* spp as part of normal aging.[4] However, lipid deposits in the central cornea typically occur in reptiles on a high fat diet.[4,11] Therefore, animals developing corneal lipid deposits should undergo diet assessment and be evaluated for hyperlipidemia. Diet changes, if needed, should be implemented and may improve corneal clarity.

Hypovitaminosis A

Commonly seen in chelonians, lack of dietary vitamin A causes squamous metaplasia of the orbital glands, ducts, and conjunctiva.[27] As a result, keratinous debris accumulates on the ducts and tears cannot be produced or reach the ocular surface. Without the protective, nutritive, and lubricating properties of the tear film, keratitis, blepharitis, and conjunctivitis result, often with profound adnexal edema. In severe cases, the palpebral fissure will close and secondary bacterial infection can occur.[28] Clinical signs may be more profound in chelonians compared with lizards due to the large size of their tear glands.[11] It is important to remember that epithelium in other organs can also undergo metaplasia with potentially fatal results. Clinical signs in combination with a thorough clinical history are often sufficient to support the diagnosis and response to treatment confirms it. In cases that fail to respond to treatment, biopsy with histologic analysis is useful for diagnosis.[4,11]

For treatment, if animals are still eating, a diet change is recommended such as commercial trout pellets supplemented with cod liver oil.[4] Early cases may be reversed with this change. Later in the disease, animals can be supplemented with parenteral vitamin A weekly until resolution.[4,29] Care must be taken in treatment dosing in order to prevent iatrogenic hypervitaminosis A.[11] Topical antibiotic ointment should be used for lubricating properties and to control secondary bacterial keratoconjunctivitis when cytology reveals heterophils or bacteria.[11,29] Lizards can also be affected (see the earlier section).

Miscellaneous causes

Fungal keratitis and exudative conjunctivitis were reported in a free-ranging Gopher tortoise secondary to traumatic injury followed by infection with *Aspergillus* and *Curvularia* spp.[30] The infection resolved following 2 months of topical miconazole administration.

CROCODILIANS
Anatomy

Unlike other reptiles, crocodilians have a more mobile upper eyelid and the tarsal plate is bony instead of cartilaginous.[6,7] The lower eyelid is less mobile and lacks a tarsal plate. Crocodilians have a large nictitating membrane controlled by the pyramidalis muscle. Although this group possesses both a Harderian gland and a lacrimal gland, they differ from lizards in typically having 3 to 8 lacrimal canaliculi that join to form the lacrimal duct. The saltwater crocodile has a single lacrimal canaliculus.[6] The cornea is thin with a thin epithelium and Descemet's membrane, thick endothelium, and no Bowman's membrane.[6]

Ocular Surface Diseases

Conjunctivitis

An outbreak of chlamydiosis resulted in fatal hepatitis and exudative conjunctivitis with fibrin deposits under the nictitating membrane in juvenile and hatchling Indo-pacific crocodiles in a farm in Papua New Guinea.[31] Diagnosis was made on post mortem identification of chlamydial colonies in liver tissue. Animal quarantine and treatment with tetracycline rapidly reduced animal losses. The source of the infection was introduction of stressed, wild-caught juveniles that likely were displaying recrudescence of chronic infection. This report highlights the importance of biosecurity when introducing new animals to a captive group.[11]

Corneal trauma

Reports of corneal and adnexal injuries in populations of farmed American alligators and wild American crocodiles suggest overcrowding is to blame.[3,32] In the population of crocodiles, environmental pollutants may have played a role in clinical signs; however, the presence of unilateral disease made this less likely.[32]

SNAKES
Anatomy

All snakes lack eyelids and instead protect the globe by means of a fixed, transparent spectacle, similar to some lizards described earlier.[6–8] Scales surround the spectacle and, in some animals, may partially overlap it. Snakes lack a nictitating membrane.

The spectacle is composed of multiple layers, the detailed anatomy of which has been recently described.[33,34] The spectacle surface is believed to be insensitive but recent work has shown deeper layers to contain nerve fibers, the function of which are unknown at this time.[33] The spectacle contains a dense vascular network that is normally invisible but becomes apparent with inflammation.[4,33,35] The keratinized surface of the spectacle is shed during ecdysis.[36] During this time, spectacle vascularity increases, fluid builds between the new and old surface, and the eye seems bluish. The spectacle clears again just before shedding.[28] The cornea is not attached to the spectacle but they are instead separated by a subspectacular space (also known as intraconjunctival space), making the globe free to move below the spectacle.[6]

Because of its design, the spectacle is a physical barrier and prevents topical medications from reaching the cornea and remainder of the globe. The snake cornea differs from lizards in that it is relatively large, contains a thin, single-layer epithelium, lacks Bowman's membrane, and has a very thin Descemet's membrane.

The anatomy of the ophidian lacrimal apparatus has been extensively studied.[6,37] Snakes typically lack a lacrimal gland and instead have a comparatively large Harderian gland that secretes tears into the subspectacular space. Tears drain through the lacrimal duct via a single opening in the ventromedial aspect of the subspectacular space. The duct takes 1 of 3 paths to open on the roof of the mouth in close proximity to the duct opening of the vomeronasal organ.[37]

Ocular Surface Diseases

Spectacle trauma

Abrasions or damage to the spectacle occur naturally given the spectacle serves a protective function. With excessive trauma, loss of spectacle clarity can result. Species that feed on live prey may be more at risk for damage; therefore, feeding live prey should be avoided when possible. Other causes include inappropriate husbandry conditions, dysecdysis, chemical exposure, parasites, and inappropriate treatment for retained spectacles.[4,38] Spectacle damage should be assessed by full ophthalmic examination. Deeper defects are more likely associated with improper husbandry or disease as opposed to normal wear and tear.

Secondary bacterial or fungal infection of deeper lesions can occur, especially if the surface epithelium is lost.[4] Cytology and culture can be useful if infection is suspected. Ophthalmic dyes such as rose bengal or fluorescein stain are not useful for spectacles. Occasionally, enclosure substrate can be lodged in the spectacle following trauma.

In most cases, the damaged tissue is shed and replaced by new surface, restoring a clear appearance. Treatment consists of topical antibiotic (ophthalmic or dermal preparations) application, provided the wounds are not full-thickness through the spectacle. Avoid using steroid preparations because they can promote secondary infection (especially fungal) or possibly delay healing.[4] Husbandry problems, such as low humidity, should be identified and corrected. Foreign material embedded in the spectacle should be removed with the aid of an operating microscope to help avoid granuloma formation or excessive inflammation.[6]

Loss of all or a portion of the spectacle can result in keratitis, corneal ulceration, panophthalmitis, and ultimately loss of vision.[4,38,39] Subsequent corneal ulceration and possibly infection can lead to scarring, permanent vision loss, and even phthisis bulbi.[4] Complete spectacle loss most often occurs when the normal spectacle is removed after being incorrectly diagnosed as retained.[38]

Treatment of partial or complete spectacle avulsion includes topical lubricant and antibiotic use, placement of a trimmed soft contact lens over the area, or use of graft material.[4,39] Recent work on spectacle healing suggests that full-thickness defects less than 25% of the total spectacular area can heal without incident in 3 months and result in a clear visual axis provided a proteinaceous plug properly forms in the defect.[40] That being said, these defects were surgically created and the outcome of other types of penetrating trauma or spectacle loss is uncertain and likely associated with more complications.[40]

Infection of the spectacle
As the spectacle is dermal in nature, it can become infected directly or through spread from adjacent skin. Most infections result from poor animal husbandry.[3,4,38] Infection can be bacterial or more often fungal.[41] Diagnosis is through cytology and culture with sensitivity testing. Treatment involves use of suitable topical and/or systemic antimicrobial agents and in some severe cases may require incision into and/or debridement of the spectacle.[4] Prognosis is better when infections are diagnosed and treated early because infection can progress to penetrate through the spectacle.[4]

Subspectacular abscess
Infection between the spectacle and cornea can occur and is one of the more common ophthalmic problems encountered in spectacled reptiles.[42] Routes of infection include penetrating trauma, hematogenous spread, or ascending from the mouth via the lacrimal duct.[4] Therefore, clinical signs can be unilateral or bilateral depending on the cause. In one study, 77% of cases were unilateral.[42] Clinical signs include a cloudy, white or yellow appearance to the spectacle with or without spectacle distortion. Facial or oral swelling may also be present based on the cause.[42] Diagnosis is made based on clinical signs and analysis of subspectacular fluid. Affected animals should undergo complete physical examination and husbandry analysis to identify the cause. CBC with or without blood culture can be performed to rule out septicemia.

Although some cases may resolve on their own, therapy typically involves partial spectaculectomy through meticulous excision of a 30° wedge of inferior spectacle to allow drainage of caseous material.[3,29,43] In addition, the animal should be anesthetized and placed under an operating microscope for ideal visualization of the narrow space. Damage to the cornea and globe are possible, even in experienced hands. Exudate samples should be collected for cytology and culture/sensitivity. Isolation of various bacterial species,[3,42] including *Pseudomonas* sp, *Proteus* sp, *Providencia rettgeri*, and *Staphylococcus* sp, fungus,[44] and nematodes[45] have been reported. The subspectacular space can then be gently flushed of exudate and treated with antibiotic solution.[3,4,29,43] Concurrent treatment of any systemic condition is vital to resolution of ocular disease. A recent retrospective study suggests resolution is likely with appropriate treatment but recurrence is possible.[42]

Pseudobuphthalmos
Blockage of the nasolacrimal duct can result in impaired drainage and subsequent buildup of tears within the subspectacular space. Clinical signs include buildup of clear or slightly cloudy fluid under a bulging spectacle. With time, the fluid can become opaque due to secondary infection, making differentiation between subspectacular abscess and pseudobuphthalmos sometimes difficult. Lacrimal duct occlusion can occur congenitally, from compression due to a tumor or granuloma or from stomatitis or subspectacular infection.[3,5,29,46,47] Diagnosis is made via observation of subspectacular space distention by clear to slightly turbid fluid on slit lamp examination.

Spontaneous resolution has been reported.[48] If signs fail to resolve on their own, partial spectaculectomy as described earlier may be performed.[4,28,46] If too small a piece is removed, recurrence is likely; however, keratitis or secondary infection can result if too large a piece is removed.[4,40,46] Attempts should be made to restore nasolacrimal duct patency when possible and treatment of any concurrent infection should be performed. Alternatively, rerouting of the lacrimal drainage via conjuntivoralostomy has been described with some success.[4,5,38] Resolution with surgical therapy is possible but recurrence has been reported.[5,42,46] Flagellates have been found in subspectacular exudate, the significance of which is unknown and may occur incidentally due to incision of spectacle vessels during surgery.[5]

Parasites
Ectoparasites such as mites (*Ophionyssus* spp and others) or ticks can be found in the sulcus depression where the scales meet the spectacle.[4,29] Diagnosis is made via visualization of the organisms, sometimes aided by slit lamp examination and manual flushing of the sulcus with balanced salt solution or eye wash. Parasitic infections commonly result from poor husbandry and can lead to retained spectacle. Therefore, treatment includes analysis for and correction of husbandry problems. Ticks can be manually removed. Mites can be treated with application of a thin film of olive oil, using a pyrethroid mite spray, or flushing the spectacle sulcus with a small volume of ivermectin followed a short time later by copious flushing of the ocular surface.[4,28] The cage can also be treated using dichlorvos.[28,29] Transdermal absorption of ivermectin is possible.

Retained spectacle
The most commonly diagnosed ocular problem in snakes is retained spectacle, defined as a failure of the old spectacle surface to shed during ecdysis.[4,42] Most cases result from poor husbandry and low environmental humidity. Dehydration, systemic illness, mite infestation, skin disease, and spectacle scarring can also

result in retention.[28] If the retained spectacle is not removed, several spectacles can accumulate, impairing vision and possibly affecting the animal's ability or willingness to feed.

Diagnosis must involve more than failing to find spectacles when examining the slough. Slit lamp examination can allow visualization of a thickened spectacle with extra layers. With enough accumulated retained spectacles, the change can be grossly visible. Occasionally, retained skin around the eye or leading to the spectacle makes the diagnosis easier.[11] Proper diagnosis is imperative before treatment is attempted because iatrogenic damage can occur to the spectacle if manual removal is inappropriately attempted. When in doubt, wait until after the next shed to confirm the diagnosis before performing any treatment.[4]

After confirming a spectacle is retained, first perform conservative treatment because it is safest. Increasing environmental humidity by misting or soaking the snake can be effective as can topical application of artificial tears or other ophthalmic lubricating ointment. One can also provide a sheet of wetted paper in the vivarium against which the snake can rub itself.[11] This will promote natural shedding during the next ecdysis. If unsuccessful, such as may occur with previous spectacle trauma and scarring, the retained spectacle can be loosened with topical application of acetylcysteine and gently removed, preferably using a wet cotton swab, taking extreme caution to avoid damaging the cornea.[4,11,28] Forceps should not be used to remove the spectacle by force unless the animal is anesthetized and under an operating microscope to ensure only the retained spectacle is removed.[11]

Miscellaneous causes of ocular surface disease

A case report described a ball python that developed anorexia, lethargy, corneal opacification, and excessive shedding and then died. Necropsy and histologic examination revealed corneal ulceration and keratoconjunctivitis in addition to epidermal changes similar to those seen with mammalian sunburn. Investigation revealed the owner had just installed "high-output" ultraviolet B lamps in the enclosure. Removal of the new lamps resulted in resolution of clinical signs in all surviving animals.[49]

Reports of tumors of the reptilian eye are rare but bilateral keratoacanthoma of the spectacle was reported in a Boa constrictor.[50] The animal had a history of poor husbandry, depression, anorexia, and dysecdysis.

SUMMARY

Reptiles can have significant variation in their ocular anatomy; therefore, consulting the literature to prepare oneself for what is normal is extremely beneficial before examining any animals. When literature on that specific species is unavailable, reading up on other members of that family or order can still be helpful. Proper restraint is key to success and prior preparation is helpful to remain efficient and minimize animal stress. Many ocular surface diseases result from improper husbandry. Therefore, obtaining a thorough history including source, diet, housing, and cleaning practices can be helpful in elucidating the cause of ocular changes. Remember that topical antimicrobial treatment is not possible in animals with an intact spectacle. Much remains to be learned about the reptile eye, so please remember to contribute to the literature when possible with your own cases and clinical experiences.

REFERENCES

1. Girling S. Reptile and amphibian handling and chemical restraint. In: Veterinary nursing of exotic pets. Sussex (England): John Wiley & Sons; 2013. p. 272 86.

2. Hernandez-Divers SJ. Diagnostic techniques. In: Mader DR, editor. Reptile medicine and surgery. 2nd edition. St Louis (MO): Elsevier; 2006. p. 490–532.
3. Millichamp NJ, Jacobson ER, Wolf ED. Disease of the eye and ocular adnexae in reptiles. J Am Vet Med Assoc 1983;183(11):1205–12.
4. Lawton MPC. Reptilian ophthalmology. In: Mader DR, editor. Reptile medicine and surgery. 2nd edition. St Louis (MO): Elsevier; 2006. p. 323–42.
5. Millichamp NJ, Jacobson ER, Dziezyc J. Conjunctivoralostomy for treatment of an occluded lacrimal duct in a blood python. J Am Vet Med Assoc 1986;189(9): 1136–8.
6. Underwood G. The eye. In: Gans C, Parsons TS, editors. Biology of the reptilia, vol. 2B. London: Academic Press; 1970. p. 1–97.
7. Duke-Elder S. The eyes of reptiles. In: Duke-Elder S, editor. The eye in evolution (System of Ophthalmology, vol. 1). London: Kimpton; 1958. p. 353–96.
8. Walls GL. The vertebrate eye and its adaptive radiation. Bloomfield Hills (MI): Cranbrook Institute of Science; 1942.
9. Williams DL, MacGregor S, Sainsbury AW. Evaluation of bacteria isolated from infected eyes of captive, non-domestic animals. Vet Rec 2000;146(18):515–8.
10. Cooper JE, McClelland MH, Needham JR. An eye infection in laboratory lizards associated with an Aeromonas sp. Lab Anim 1980;14(2):149–51.
11. Williams DL. The reptile eye. In: Ophthalmology of exotic pets. Ames (IA): Wiley-Blackwell; 2012. p. 159–96.
12. Boyer TH. Common problems of leopard geckos. Proceedings of the Association of Reptilian and Amphibian Veterinarians Conference. Indianapolis, IN, 2013.
13. Miller EA, Green SL, Otto GM, et al. Suspected hypovitaminosis A in a colony of captive green anoles (Anolis carolinensis). Contemp Top Lab Anim Sci 2001; 40(2):18–20.
14. Coke RL, Couillard NK. Ocular biology and diseases of Old World chameleons. Vet Clin North Am Exot Anim Pract 2002;5(2):275–85.
15. Dunson WA. Salt glands in reptiles. In: Gans C, Dawson WR, editors. Biology of the reptilia, vol. 5. London: Academic Press; 1976. p. 413–45.
16. Abel JH, Ellis RA. Histochemical and electron microscopic observations on the salt secreting lacrimal glands of marine turtles. Am J Anat 1966;118(2):337–57.
17. König D. Der vordere Augenabschnitt der Schildkröten und die Funktion seiner Muskulatur. Jena Z Naturw 1935;69:223–84.
18. Northmore DP, Granda AM. Ocular dimensions and schematic eyes of freshwater and sea turtles. Vis Neurosci 1991;7(6):627–35.
19. Brown MB, Mclaughlin GS, Klein PA, et al. Upper respiratory tract disease in the gopher tortoise is caused by Mycoplasma agassizii. J Clin Microbiol 1999;37: 2262–9.
20. Feldman SH, Wimsatt J, Marchang RE, et al. A novel mycoplasma detected in association with upper respiratory disease syndrome in free ranging eastern box turtles (Terrapene carolina carolina) in Virginia. J Wildl Dis 2006;42(2):279–89.
21. Platt TR. Helminth parasites of the western painted turtle, Chrysemys picta belli (Gray), including Neopolystoma elizabethae n. sp. (Monogenea: Polystomatidae), a parasite of the conjunctival sac. J Parasitol 2000;86(4):815–8.
22. Pichelin S. The taxonomy and biology of the Polystomatidae (Monogenea) in Australian freshwater turtles (Chelidae, Pleurodira). J Nat Hist 1995;29(6): 1345–81.
23. Jacobson ER, Clubb S, Gaskin JM, et al. Herpesviruslike infection in Argentine tortoises. J Am Vet Med Assoc 1985;187:1227–9.

24. Jacobson ER, Gaskin JM, Roelke M, et al. Conjunctivitis, tracheitis and pneumonia associated with herpesvirus infection in green sea turtles. J Am Vet Med Assoc 1986;189(9):1020–3.

25. Lackovich JK, Brown DR, Homer BL, et al. Association of herpesvirus with fibropapillomatosis of the green turtle Chelonia mydas and the loggerhead turtle Caretta caretta in Florida. Dis Aquat Organ 1999;37(2):89–97.

26. Brooks DE, Ginn PE, Miller TR, et al. Ocular fibropapillomas of green turtles (Chelonia mydas). Vet Pathol 1994;31:335–9.

27. Elkan E, Zwart P. The ocular disease of young terrapins caused by vitamin A deficiency. Vet Pathol 1967;4(3):201–22.

28. Kern TJ, Colitz CMH. Exotic animal ophthalmology. In: Gelatt KN, Gilger BC, Kern TJ, editors. Veterinary ophthalmology. 5th edition. Ames (IA): Wiley-Blackwell; 2013. p. 1750–819.

29. Millichamp N. Exotic animal ophthalmology. In: Gelatt KN, editor. Veterinary ophthalmology. 2nd edition. Philadelphia: Lea & Febiger; 1991. p. 680–705.

30. Myers DA, Isaza R, Ben-Shlomo G, et al. Fungal keratitis in a Gopher tortoise (Gopherus polyphemus). J Zoo Wildl Med 2009;40(3):579–82.

31. Huchzermeyer F, Langelet E, Putterill J. An outbreak of chlamydiosis in farmed Indopacific crocodiles (Crocodylus porosus). J S Afr Vet Assoc 2008;79(2): 99–100.

32. Rainwater TR, Millichamp NJ, Barrantes LD, et al. Ocular disease in American crocodiles (Crocodylus acutus) in Costa Rica. J Wildl Dis 2011;47(2):415–26.

33. Da Silva MA, Heegaard S, Wang T, et al. The spectacle of the ball python (Python regius): a morphological description. J Morphol 2014;275(5):489–96.

34. Hollingsworth SR, Holmberg BJ, Strunk A, et al. Comparison of ophthalmic measurements obtained via high-frequency ultrasound imaging in four species of snakes. Am J Vet Res 2007;68:1111–4.

35. Mead AW. Vascularity in the reptilian spectacle. Invest Ophthalmol 1976;15(7): 587–91.

36. Maderson PFA. Histological changes in the epidermis of snakes during the sloughing cycle. J Zool 1965;146:98–113.

37. Souza NM, Maggs DJ, Park SA, et al. Gross, histologic, and micro-computed tomographic anatomy of the lacrimal system of snakes. Vet Ophthalmol 2015; 18(Suppl 1):15–22.

38. Lawton MPC. Introduction to reptilian ophthalmology. Proceedings of the Association of Reptilian and Amphibian Veterinarians Annual Conference. Kansas City, MO, 1998. p. 115–8.

39. Divers SJ, Lawton MPC. The use of lyophilised skin grafts for the treatment of integumental disease in birds and reptiles. Proceedings of the British Small Animal Veterinary Association Congress 2000.

40. Maas AK, Paul-Murphy J, Kumaresan-Lampman S, et al. Spectacle wound healing in the royal python (Python regius). J Herpetol Med Surg 2010;20(1):29–36.

41. Cheatwood JO, Jacobson ER, May PG, et al. An outbreak of fungal dermatitis and stomatitis in a free-ranging population of pigmy rattlesnakes (Sistrurus miliarius barbouri) in Florida. J Wildl Dis 2003;39:329–37.

42. Hausmann JC, Hollingsworth SR, Hawkins MG, et al. Distribution and outcome of ocular lesions in snakes examined at a veterinary teaching hospital: 67 cases (1985-2010). J Am Vet Med Assoc 2013;243(2):252–60.

43. Miller WW. Subspectacular abscess in a Burmese python. Auburn Vet 1986; 41:19–21.

44. Zwart P, Verwer M, Vries GD, et al. Fungal infection of the eyes of the snake Epicrates chenchria maurus: enucleation under Halothane narcosis. J Small Anim Pract 1973;14(12):773–9.
45. Hausmann JC, Mans C, Dreyfus J, et al. Subspectacular nematodiasis caused by a novel Serpentirhabdias species in ball pythons (Python regius). J Comp Pathol 2015;152(2–3):260–4.
46. Cullen CL, Wheler C, Grahn BH. Diagnostic ophthalmology. Bullous spectaculopathy in a king snake. Can Vet J 2000;41(4):327–8.
47. Sabater M, Perez M. Congenital ocular and adnexal disorders in reptiles. Vet Ophthalmol 2013;16(1):47–55.
48. Ensley PK, Anderson MP, Bacon JP. Ophthalmic disorders in three snakes. J Zoo Anim Med 1978;9:57–9.
49. Gardiner DW, Baines FM, Pandher K. Photodermatitis and photokeratoconjunctivitis in a ball python (Python regius) and a blue-tongue skink (Tiliqua spp.). J Zoo Wildl Med 2009;40(4):757–66.
50. Hardon T, Fledelius B, Heegaard S. Keratoacanthoma of the spectacle in a Boa constrictor. Vet Ophthalmol 2007;10(5):320–2.

Moving?

Make sure your subscription moves with you!

To notify us of your new address, find your **Clinics Account Number** (located on your mailing label above your name), and contact customer service at:

Email: **journalscustomerservice-usa@elsevier.com**

800-654-2452 (subscribers in the U.S. & Canada)
314-447-8871 (subscribers outside of the U.S. & Canada)

Fax number: **314-447-8029**

**Elsevier Health Sciences Division
Subscription Customer Service
3251 Riverport Lane
Maryland Heights, MO 63043**

*To ensure uninterrupted delivery of your subscription, please notify us at least 4 weeks in advance of move.